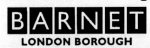
Please return/renew this item by the
last date shown to avoid a charge.
Books may also be renewed by phone
and Internet. May not be renewed if
required by another reader.

www.libraries.barnet.gov.uk

BARNET
LONDON BOROUGH

TAKING THE MEDICINE

By the same author

Digging up the Dead: Uncovering the Life and Times
of an Extraordinary Surgeon

TAKING THE MEDICINE

A Short History of Medicine's Beautiful Idea
and our Difficulty Swallowing It

Druin Burch

Chatto & Windus
LONDON

Druin Burch has asserted his right under the Copyright, Designs and Patents Act 1988 to be identified as the author of this work

This book is sold subject to the condition that it shall not, by way of trade or otherwise, be lent, resold, hired out, or otherwise circulated without the publisher's prior consent in any form of binding or cover other than that in which it is published and without a similar condition, including this condition, being imposed on the subsequent purchaser

First published in Great Britain in 2009 by
Chatto & Windus
Random House, 20 Vauxhall Bridge Road,
London SW1V 2SA

www.rbooks.co.uk

Addresses for companies within The Random House Group Limited can be found at:
www.randomhouse.co.uk/offices.htm

The Random House Group Limited Reg. No. 954009

A CIP catalogue record for this book is available from the British Library

ISBN 9780701182786

The Random House Group Limited supports The Forest Stewardship Council (FSC), the leading international forest certification organisation. All our titles that are printed on Greenpeace-approved FSC-certified paper carry the FSC logo. Our paper-procurement policy can be found at www.rbooks.co.uk/environment

Typeset by SX Composing DTP, Rayleigh
Printed and bound in Great Britain by
CPI Mackays, Chatham ME5 8TD

To Theodore John Burch, who didn't help at all

Contents

Prologue

Few things are more frightening than standing over someone with a very large needle, the intention of plunging it into their neck for their own benefit, and no previous experience of success.

I am not talking about the little needles you use to give drugs, or the slightly bigger ones for blood transfusions. I mean the large and long pieces of sharpened steel that are used for making entry holes into people's bodies.

The process is meant to be straightforward. You lie the patient flat, or tilt the bed backwards so that the head is below the feet and the blood vessels of the head and neck engorge. You clean the skin, put sterile drapes all around the neck (which means covering over the face) and inject some local anaesthetic around the jugular vein. Then, gloved and gowned, with a mask on your face and a cap on your head, you feel in the neck for a pulse. The heat of all the extra clothes makes you sweat. You find a pulse, then pause for a second to make sure it is not your own. Under your fingers, now, is the patient's carotid artery, each pulse taking a beat's worth of blood towards the brain. In most people the vein you need lies just to the outside of this pulsation.

Keeping your fingers on the pulse, you grab a very large needle attached to a small syringe. The vein you are after is deep beneath the skin. You cannot see it or feel it. The needle might pass through it or miss it entirely. It can pierce the artery, where the blood squirts along

1

under high pressure, or it can pass through and puncture the top of a lung. It can make a hole in the windpipe or cut through important nerves.

You grab the syringe in one hand and, carefully, put the end of the needle on the skin of the patient's neck, next to your fingers. The tip is bevelled and sharp, not a round 'O' but, seen in profile as you are seeing it now, a piercing 'V'. If you are lucky the patient is not moving their head, or twitching, and you are not nervously aware of how easy it is to plunge the needle through the thin protection of your surgical gloves and into your own hand.

'You may feel some slight pushing now,' you say, hoping it sounds more convincing to the patient.

My education in placing these needles began on a ward that was unusually organised about monitoring it. That was because two months before my arrival, a doctor tried the procedure and failed. He put his needle into the carotid artery. When he took the syringe off the end of the needle, just to make sure, the blood spurted out with enough force to spatter its way across the length of the room. Hitting the carotid is reasonably common. You press hard enough for long enough and the bleeding usually stops.

The doctor then tried on the other side of the patient's neck, where he made the same mistake. Withdrawing, he pressed again to encourage the bleeding to stop.

The patient's neck swelled. Over each side there was a bulge of blood. It was contained within her flesh, not pouring uncontrollably onto the floor. The pressure grew in her neck, the two tomato-like swellings squashing the structures around them. The patient began to struggle for breath. The two internal bleeds, not much more than big bruises, pressed on her windpipe. They crushed it. She died.

Medical interventions are dangerous. Things sometimes go wrong, no matter how careful you are. It is easy to understand when looking at a large needle, somehow harder when it comes to a pill. Sharp edges are not required to make something dangerous. I have given clot-busting drugs to people having heart attacks, then seen them bleed so rapidly into their tongue that it has swollen and choked them. Others have collapsed with strokes, the drugs saving their hearts at the same time as making them bleed torrentially into their own brains. Even when the deaths are not so dramatic, they are as real. Drugs can do their damage unobtrusively, scarcely noticed. A little more confusion than someone normally suffers, a slight step forwards in the crumbling of old age. Someone with cancer beginning to bleed internally, vomiting up their own blood. When you have been expecting something bad to happen, it is easy to overlook the fact that a pill may have hurried it along.

There are also the errors of omission. A doctor, remembering that two of his patients have bled to death from aspirin over the last month, becomes wary of giving it to others. The bleeds stick in his memory, nagging at him. The purpose of the aspirin is to fend off strokes and heart attacks, yet the patients carry on having them whether they are on the drug or not. Those few people who die spectacularly from blood loss are memorable. The many others whose heart attacks and strokes happen a little bit later, a little less often: they are less vivid. So the doctor slips in his habits, and the errors of omission happen in obscurity. When an old man clutches his chest and collapses, as all his family knew he one day might, it is easy to ignore the drugs that he was *not* on. Yet these deaths, too, are side effects of medical dangers.

You would think that doctors, aware of these dangers, know what they are doing and that seeking medical advice is a *good* thing. Most of the time you'd be right, but only recently. Doctors, for most of human history, have killed their patients far more often than they have saved them. Their drugs and their advice have been poisonous. They have been sincere, well-meaning and murderous. This book is

3

about medicine's bleak past, and the methods it learnt in order to improve.

Using a handful of common drugs – opium, aspirin, quinine and a few others – I want to show how the *way* in which people have thought about medicine has determined their success. Different treatments tell different tales. Those collected together here share a common theme. Their story is about the importance of how you try to answer questions about the human body, about what makes it healthy or sick, and how surprisingly difficult it can be to tell the difference.

Most histories of medicine are strikingly odd. They treat their subject as though it was a matter of perspective, of judgement, of opinion. Roy Porter's *The Greatest Benefit to Mankind* is the best of the comprehensive modern histories. In his introduction Porter apologises for focusing on the people who made advances, disliking the idea of a '"great docs" history which celebrated the triumphal progress of medicine from ignorance through error to science'. Porter was abashed about the extent to which he concentrated on the West. He did so, he explained, only because Western approaches became so culturally successful. 'Its dominance', he says, meaning that of Western medicine, 'has increased because it is perceived, by societies and the sick, to "work" uniquely well, at least for many major classes of disorders.'

Why should Porter put the word *work* in quotation marks?

Historians treat medicine the way they do politics and society and art. The Egyptians used ostrich egg poultices for open skull fractures, just as they mummified their dead and built pyramids for them. All these activities, for historians, fit into the system of beliefs that defined what it was to be an ancient Egyptian. And to the extent that another culture's medicine is as much a part of who people are as their religion, these historians are right. Porter's brilliantly written history contains thrilling accounts of the remedies used by the Egyptians, the Greeks, the Romans, the Victorian English.

Did their medicines save lives, cure ills, and offer comfort to them in their distress? Here the historians are less helpful. They will not tell you. Their interest is in the way the therapies reflect the beliefs of particular cultures. Porter's interest, like that of most historians, is in the cultural relativity of medicine. What may be a cure to my eyes could be a poison to yours. Each society's 'diagnostic arts and therapeutic interventions', Porter says, are as valid as any others. He focuses on Western ones because of their worldwide popularity. This is the traditional view of medical history, in which medical systems war with each other like religions, battling it out for the hearts of the faithful.

Yet medicines are not like poems, the different virtues of pills and potions as capable of endless debate as odes and sonnets. Our bodies are the bodies of the Egyptians that came before us, and the Sumerians that came before them. We have the same organs and the same construction. The cancers and infectious diseases and hazards of accident and age have changed a little over the millennia, but not a great deal. Histories of medicine give readers a rich feeling for the vast array of drugs that the Greeks and Romans, the Chinese and Indians and eighteenth-century French, possessed. They provide a clear account of what people believed they were doing, but almost none at all of whether they were right.

Suffering from cancer, did a patient get better treatment under medieval French physicians than under the Egyptian doctor Imhotep? Struck down with pneumonia, was someone better off being bled for it by the Greeks, the Romans, the Renaissance Italians, the Revolutionary Americans or the best minds of nineteenth-century medicine from Harvard to Heidelberg? The answer is that it made no difference. The rationales varied, but not the effects. The Greeks had an explanation for why taking 4 pints of blood away would help someone with a chest infection. George Washington's doctors had their own explanations. In terms of understanding the cultures of the two civilisations who held those views, the differences between their explanations are interesting. Relative to the effects of blood loss on a sick human being they matter not at all.

The Egyptians had complicated ideas about how the body worked and they believed that lettuce was a drug that caused lust. What happened a thousand years later, in the classical civilisations of Athens and Rome? Thomas Dormandy's recent history of pain is long and entertaining. When he gets to the Greeks and the Romans he comments that 'the garden lettuce gathered when young and tender had an established reputation as a mollifier of grief. But it could also encourage frenzy.' Could the lettuce have changed from the days of Egypt? Could human physiology? Should we be wary of salads?

On the last day of 1664, Samuel Pepys wrote in his diary of his unusually good health over the previous months. 'I am at a great loss to know whether it be my Hare's fote, or taking every morning a pill of Turpentine, or my having left off the wearing of a gowne.' Whatever the cause, it was none of those three. We are still at a loss for many things, frequently including physical explanations, but we have progressed since 1664. Medical progress is real, and it comes from realising that some medical theories are more useful than others. Pepys's beliefs were sincere, but they were wrong.

The United Nations Children's Fund started monitoring global child deaths in 1960. In 2007 they reported that for the first time deaths dropped below 10 million a year. Over the same period the number of children in the world rose. In 1960 20 million died each year. In 2007 the number was 9.7 million. The reason for the success was that some poor countries became a little less poor, meaning better food and housing and sanitation, while vaccinations and vitamins and mosquito nets helped save millions of children's lives. Progress relies on understanding that some medical treatments really do 'work'.

I never intended to save any lives. It was sort of an accident, arranged chiefly with a view to extending my sporting life. A time spent in genetic research failed – I found the pipette too dull a companion and the statistics too frightening – yet the outside world was not attractive. I could not understand the rush of my colleagues towards the City of London. That meant suits and rigid working lives, not to mention very little opportunity to do any sport. The thought of a 'proper job' was equivalent in my mind with middle age. My mental world was divided up into sport and non-sport, and it was the first that I wished to live in.

So with these hidden motives, I applied for medical school. My interview preparation was largely non-existent. 'What if they ask you why you want to be a doctor?' suggested a friend. 'They won't ask me that,' I explained. 'Why would anyone ask such a dull question? They'll only get identical answers about liking science and wanting to help people.'

'Why do you want to be a doctor?' they asked me.

Whatever I said has long passed from my memory. Probably the examiners were not even listening. To this day I think it was a bad question. Medicine seemed reasonably interesting and reasonably honourable, but I did not have the first idea how I might one day feel practising it. How can you, other than by giving it a go?

Medical school went smoothly. My surgical tutor wrote me the kindest of possible reports. 'I have not met this student,' he recorded, some months after I was allocated to his weekly tutorials. 'But I understand his rowing has improved enormously.' It had. I never did turn up to any of my surgical teaching and the surgeon, whom I later discovered to be eminent, passed me without problems.

One summer I needed an excuse to stay on during the vacation and train. A helpful tutor, hoping my plans might represent some academic enthusiasm, helped me win a small grant to pursue medical history during the summer. So, after mornings going up and down the Thames, I spent the bulk of each sunny day sitting in an old library. I sat there reading until the heat of the day softened into gentle warmth, and then I went out rowing again. It was perfect. I read about the practice of medicine during the nineteenth and early twentieth centuries. It seemed very civilised, in many ways, except that the treatments were laughable. Leeches were popular, along with a range of other interventions that also shortened people's lives. I found it remarkable that no one at the time noticed.

When the summer was over (and winter training properly begun) we learnt about heart attacks. One of my books told me that you used a drug called lignocaine, but it wasn't mentioned in the lectures. I put my hand up and asked about it.

'We don't use that these days,' I was told.

'But my book says it saves lives.'

'Not any more. Nowadays it kills people.'

The lecturer was echoing a famous exchange from Molière, often quoted in medical journals:

GÉRONTE: It seems to me you are locating them wrongly: the heart is on the left and the liver is on the right.
SGANARELLE: Yes, in the old days that was so, but we have changed all that, and we now practise medicine by a completely new method.

How could something save lives one year and cost them the next? The days of leeches began to seem not so very far away. Now I noticed other contradictions in my textbooks. One said that amphetamines were good for helping students to concentrate, and that family doctors were happy to prescribe them. Another explained that antidepressants made people commit suicide. A third said that pregnant women should drink Guinness. The fourth stated that bed-rest saved lives, while the fifth was confident it cost them. On the wards, senior doctors in the mornings told you to avoid certain things at all costs, while others in the afternoon declared the same treatments to be essential. Professors disagreed over whether people had infections, heart attacks, cancers and strokes – and then argued that their opponent's treatments were likely to be disastrous.

Around this time we were introduced to something called 'evidence-based medicine'. Truth, it suggested, was not something that could be divined by the mysterious insight of experts. You developed a theory and then you tested it, and only certain types of tests were reliable.

A lot of things that seemed confusing started becoming clear. I began to understand about the leeches, and the textbooks and the professors. If someone senior and wise believed that something worked, it was not necessarily true. Even though sincere and educated and intelligent people thought a treatment was helpful, it could still be toxic.

Down by the river, things also changed. Formerly my coaches had seemed like gods, gifted with perfect understanding and total power. Any time I failed, it was clear to me that it was my fault: some limitation in myself. The coaches shared these views. No matter how certain I was of their wisdom and understanding, they were more certain still.

'I want you to keep your heart rates at 85 per cent of max. for the next hour and a half,' they said. It was the kind of thing they said quite often.

'Why?' I began to ask.

There was usually a short pause.

'Because it's the best way to improve your fitness.'

'How do you know?'

There was a longer pause.

'Because I've done it before and it worked. Because that's what the people who win the Olympics do. I know, I've trained some of them.'

'But,' I asked, 'has anyone actually done an experiment?'

Another short pause, but this time a little more threatening.

'What on earth are you talking about?'

This book is my answer.

1 Early Medicine and Opium

When our ancestors ceased to gather and hunt some ten to fifteen thousand years ago, they were making a curious choice, not least because it made them less healthy. Their diet became more restricted, and more vulnerable to a bad season affecting one or two main crops. Domestic animals brought with them lice and worms and diseases that hadn't had a crack at *Homo sapiens* until that point. Hygiene became more of a problem. You don't need to be too scrupulous about where you defecate if you are likely to move on the next day. That changed. Average lifespan, at least for a little while, went down.

What agriculture did provide (other than a steady supply of beer, which some people have seriously argued was what made it attractive to begin with) was the opportunity for acquiring wealth. Grain could be stored, workers could specialise, chiefs could rise to the top and get fat and lazy. Healers, for the first time, could really concentrate on their craft. With large agriculturally minded populations, specialised professional doctors first appeared.

The Sumerians, the earliest agricultural society we know much about, lived around six thousand years ago in what is now Iraq. They had faith in their medics. 'My son, pay attention to everything medical! . . . pay attention to everything medical!' were the words of a Sumerian matron who, in the manner of many mothers since, felt her offspring paid so little attention that she needed to repeat herself.

The Sumerians worried about 'the anxiety and intestinal disease which pursue mankind', as well as afflictions beyond the power of medicine ('A malicious wife living in the house is worse than all disease,' ran one proverb). They wrote of potions, of a doctor 'who keeps people alive, and brings them to birth' and of making 'perfect the divine powers of medicine'.

To get an idea of Sumerian medicine, we have to turn to the Egyptians. The clay tablets we have from the Sumerians contain poems, proverbs, history, religion and even a novel, but they are short on medical details. One does list a few medical ingredients – the shells of turtles, skins of snakes, thyme and milk and figs and dates – but gives no clue as to their preparation or intended uses. The Egyptians, however, inherited a great deal from the civilisation of Sumer, and we also have a better record of the specifics they offered to their sick. They were not, generally speaking, up to much.

Edwin Smith, a middle-aged adventurer from Connecticut, spent £12 in January of 1862 for two papyri. They were around three and a half thousand years old, and included knowledge handed down from long before that. They list around 160 different remedies, of which modern scholars have translated a small portion. So we know that the medical armouries of the Egyptians contained onions and watermelons and celery, as well as almonds and aniseed, dates and dill, juniper and cinnamon.

A recent historian of aspirin, Diarmuid Jeffreys, grew excited about the inclusion in this Egyptian list, as well as in that of the Sumerians, of willow. It is from willow that we originally get aspirin. It would be nice to think that this meant the Sumerians and the Egyptians were using willow in a medically effective way. They drew no distinction, however, between willow and their other ingredients. As far as they were concerned, willow was no more effective than onions or celery.

One of the papyri that Smith bought suggested mixing willow with figs, dates and beer to 'cause the heart to receive bread'. (The Egyptians used 'bread' as a synonym for all sorts of fine things. Their daily greeting for each other was a cheerful wish for 'Bread and beer!' meaning pretty much everything in life that was good.) The historian of aspirin commented that 'many of their superstitions, reasoning and treatments are based on concepts that are alien to us'. That is true, but it is not what really matters. The Egyptians considered their doctors and their medicines as being potent and effective. Records of their practices show something different. These papyri, the oldest proper medical instructions of our species, contained potions and salves and drugs whose effectiveness was a fantasy. Traditional knowledge of healing was not reliable. The first doctors in the world were frauds. This was a remarkable beginning for any profession, even more so for one that has always delighted in a special trust. For the next three and a half thousand years, little changed.

Despite it all, the world grew more populated. People began living longer. They became healthier. By the start of the twentieth century, someone lucky enough to be born in the developed part of the world could expect to live for almost three times the lifespan of their gatherer-hunter ancestor. This huge change came from having more food, better shelter and richer environments. Medicine took away more than it added.

The idea of science – the notion that theories must be tested, and that those that cannot or have not been tested are something other than facts – did not occur to the Sumerians. They had one drug, however, that worked so immediately and so obviously that they understood its effects. That drug came from the poppy, and it has stayed popular to this day.

The poppy is of the genus *Papaver*, family *Papaveraceae*, order *Ranunculales*, class *Magnoliopsida*, division *Magnoliophyta*, kingdom *Plantae* and the domain of the eukaryotes. It prefers soil that has been disturbed, by war or by the plough, and is a common sight in the Oxfordshire fields that surround my home. *Papaver rhoeas* is an annual plant, springing up in the midst of the small irregular fields of wheat and barley. It has the hairy stalk and drooping green flower bud of the *Papaver* genus, rearing up its head to the sun when its twin sepals fall and the scarlet and black petals beneath burst out for a few bright days. Other poppies have other colours: the oranges of the Californian poppy, *Platystemon californicus*, the clear yellow of the Welsh or the host of shades in which the large Iceland poppy appears.

With warm summer days the poppy's ovary swells. A fruit is formed, an upturned bell, the stigma forming a cap where the clapper should be. For a time this fruit is obviously lactiferous. Scratch it, and a white substance oozes slowly from the seed-head. Eventually, though, it dries, and the breezes blow the seeds through the capsule's pores, the plants of another year.

Growing up in the later part of the twentieth century, the poppy seemed to me to symbolise happiness. You saw them when idling in the countryside in good weather, or glimpsed them from the window of a train or a car, flashes of bright scarlet. Even the perpetual image of the Flanders fields heightened the sense of the poppy's cheerful nature. It was partly this contrast with the mud and the death all around that made it appeal so much to the troops: the way it crept into their minds like the promise of the pastoral home for which so many believed they were fighting, their memories of rural joy.

That was what the Sumerians called it: the joy plant. Their writing was cuneiform, a clumsier form of symbolism than our generally phonetic alphabet, and many of the clay tablets they used have survived. One from south of Baghdad describes how to extract the joy from the plant. You score the ripening seed-heads, and the bitter-tasting, drug-filled latex emerges. Leave it to dry and oxidise in the sun, then return and collect the brown sticky paste that results. What you have is opium.

Opium itself – the dried sap of the poppy – is a mixture of different chemicals, the most important of which we today call morphine. It is one of a class of compounds called alkaloids, many of which have pharmacological effects. Why they should do so is not fully clear, but it appears at least in part to be because many alkaloids are produced by plants specifically to have an effect on the species around them. Many make a plant (or a portion of it) unappetising to whatever insect or herbivore might be otherwise tempted to eat it. Some of these defences can occasionally become attractions, as when people seek out chilli peppers for the heat that is meant to make mammals avoid them. In a similar way the production of morphine has proved to be a successful evolutionary adaptation for the poppy. The drug binds to neurons throughout our brain and spinal cord, subduing pain and producing happiness, as well as damping down both our drive to breathe and the normal movement of our bowels. For this, as well as for the delights of its flower, people have been moved to propagate and protect the plant.

There are other ways of extracting opiates from *Papaver*, some of them simpler. Eating a poppy-seed bagel is sufficient to fail a drugs test; the stuff is in there, even if the doses are too low for you to feel. A botanist at the United States Department of Agriculture has suggested that there are significant quantities of opiates in all poppies, and that an unripe seed-head steeped in a glass of vodka could produce enough for a more than decent dose. Less than a century ago the same government department was advising farmers on planting drug poppies as a good cash crop.

If we take a drug in order to bring joy, is it a medicine? Using a drug to produce a sense of well-being does not seem 'medical' to most of us. Yet unhappiness, at least according to some, is a form of illness. So says the World Health Organisation, whose definition of health is stridently positive. Health, declares the WHO, 'is a state of complete physical, mental and social well-being and not merely the absence of disease or infirmity'. From that perspective anything that brings happiness brings health. Opium has been used since ancient times as an antidepressant drug. Sometimes we still use it medically in similar ways. I have injected people with morphine and seen their fear, their misery and terror dissolve. Was it just that they were in pain, and the pain loosened their worst feelings? Perhaps. But sometimes pain and terror and unhappiness are not separate things. Opium can treat them all.

Papaver rhoeas, the poppy of the Flanders fields, is a poor producer of useful drugs. For potency you need a poppy like *Papaver setigerum* or, even better, *Papaver somniferum*. If a field of poppies reminds most of us of summer or of war, in days gone by poppies evoked sleep and rest and forgetfulness. Poetry was rich with it. Homer sang of Helen, daughter of Zeus, preparing a draught by which Odysseus's son Telemachus might forget the pang of his absence. She 'cast a drug into the wine of which they drank to lull all pain and anger and bring forgetfulness of every sorrow'. That certainly sounds like opium, the drug that a Victorian poet described as making him feel his soul were being rubbed down with silk. Dioscorides, who wrote a five-volume textbook of pharmacology in the first century AD, thought Helen had used henbane. That is an altogether less predictable and less beatific drug and it seems unlikely, although Dioscorides, who travelled with the Roman military and almost certainly collected opium as he went, had some authority. More modern writers believe that Helen used opium, and an article in the *Bulletin of Narcotics* in 1967 even suggested that Telemachus avoided any ill-effects by virtue of being a regular user. It is not clear where in the *Odyssey* they found the authority for such a belief, but the *Bulletin of Narcotics*, perhaps, has some lingering worries about the effect of Homer on impressionable minds.

English poetry, especially in the nineteenth and twentieth centuries, was rich with the poppy. It bloomed with connotations of sleep, oblivion and mock-death – blessings all. Francis Thompson's 'The Poppy', written around 1887, today seems rather unintentionally soporific and forgettable. In 1919, though, it was regarded highly enough to make it into the *Oxford Book of English Verse*. There the poppy also hangs sleepily from Tennyson's craggy ridge, and blows in the Flanders fields of John McCrae. Isaac Rosenberg knew how a poet should keep a poppy safe, especially at break of day in the trenches:

> Poppies whose roots are in man's veins
> Drop, and are ever dropping;
> But mine in my ear is safe,
> Just a little white with the dust.

Private Rosenberg was killed at dawn on 1 April 1918, having just completed a night patrol. Oscar Wilde, in tune with his occasional declarations that he reserved his best genius for his life rather than his work, preferred wearing poppies to writing about them. The homoerotic symbolism of the poppy, particularly a floppy-petalled purple one, helped prepare the ground for war poets who needed images to describe the red wounds of fresh young men. After McCrae's 'In Flanders Fields', the poppy became the symbol of the War to End All Wars – and then of the wars after it. The symbol of oblivion became that of remembrance.

Papaver somniferum has been found in human settlements dating back six or seven thousand years. It grew widely across Europe and Asia, perhaps being domesticated in the western Mediterranean. Burials in the Murciélagos Cave in Spain, dating to around 4200 BC, were accompanied by bags of poppy seed-capsules.

The ancient Egyptians, after the fashion of the Sumerians, cultivated the poppy. They used it for many purposes, but they were clear about its medical power. In their pantheon the god Isis gave opium to Ra, the sun god, to clear up his headache. In their long list of medical treatments, the poppy was important, in some ways unique.

In Roman days, Nero was fond of the poppy. Pliny reported that the emperor used it as a way of getting rid of his enemies. Coleridge, two thousand years later, found it enthralling. 'How divine that repose is,' he said, of the dreams it brought, 'what a spot of enchantment, a green spot of fountains and flowers and trees in the very heart of a waste of sands.' His London lectures, popular enough that the world's first one-way system was created outside to handle the traffic, were based on his belief that he could only be at his most interesting to his audience if he was also at his most interesting to himself. So he stepped up to speak with no fixed ideas of his script, and opened his mouth to hear what ideas came out. Into a glass of water on the podium he poured a little laudanum, opium in alcohol, and a few drops of it were enough to colour the whole glass. As he spoke he added more, and as the talk progressed the glass grew darker.

Here was something that was unmistakably a drug. The poppy caused sleep and happiness, it relieved depression, shortness of breath and – remarkably – diarrhoea. Above all it could take away pain. Oscar Wilde, dying in the shabbiness that overtook his last years, was given morphine and opium to take away the pain of what the doctors believed to be a fatal meningitis. Towards the end, in November of 1900, they took the strange step of only pretending to give him the injections. Wilde, his mind half gone with disease, was reduced to shoving his hand into his mouth to keep from screaming. That his doctors withheld morphine was undoubtedly cruel, but it may have prolonged Wilde's life a fraction. The poppy's ability to deliver people from a feeling of suffocation is not because it helps them breathe. It does the opposite, taking away their awareness of being short of breath. That eases away people's suffering. Potentially it eases away their lives too.

Appreciation of a drug's effects does not mean that the theories used to explain them are correct. Opium, said Galen, 'is the strongest of the drugs which numb the senses and induce a deadening sleep'. Galen was a Greek living in Rome during the second century after Christ. He is the most influential doctor ever to have lived. His writings summed up the classical knowledge of the time, with a few of his own innovations thrown in. For over a thousand years after he died his beliefs were accepted as absolute truth. Despite Galen's proclaimed belief in experimentation, the bulk of his knowledge was based on insight. Galen recommended soaking opium in boiling water, then using it on a woollen sponge either up past the anus or into the nose. Both methods work, the blood supply to the rectum and the nostrils being rich, and the mucous membranes lining those body parts being thin and easily permeable. Galen possessed opium. He had other drugs that gave people diarrhoea – senna and castor oil are still used today – and ones that made them vomit or sweat. Such effects were within the capability of primitive people to discover.

Anthropologists have sworn off using the word 'primitive', worried that it implies that others have cultures that are less complex or rich than our own. They may be correct. When it comes to objective knowledge, however, the word is truthful. Galen's understanding of medicine really was primitive compared to ours, just as ours will hopefully be compared to that of our grandchildren.

What was it about these early drugs that enabled people to discover them? If something, relatively quickly, made someone vomit, sweat, hallucinate or become unconscious then you could see it. If the person's bowels or bladder behaved differently, he or she was able to tell someone about it the next day. Drugs with these effects could be pinned down by the same processes that helped people discover what was good to eat. Subtler effects, and longer time-scales, were not so easy. Many poisons which worked slowly were missed. The Romans sweetened their wine with lead. It was not obvious that the painful and lingering deaths that resulted – decades afterwards – were caused by the metal dissolved in the wine. Beneficial effects were overlooked too, if they were not immediate, dramatic and unmistakable. From the food they ate to the plants in their gardens, people were surrounded by substances containing active drugs – but they lacked the means to notice them.

This is not the impression given by standard medical histories. Roy Porter's 1997 *The Greatest Benefit to Mankind* puts it this way: '. . . after much pooh-poohing of "primitive medicine", pharmacologists studying ethnobotany now acknowledge that such lore provided healers with effective analgesics, anaesthetics, emetics, purgatives, diuretics, narcotics, cathartics, febrifuges, contraceptives and abortifacients'. Porter's list is generally accurate, yet his effect is to mislead. What, for example, did Galen possess? Emetics worked in that they made people vomit, but what conditions benefit from vomiting? Purgatives are useful for constipation but little else. In infections they serve a similar role to bleeding and emetics – helping to dehydrate and weaken patients who are already dehydrated and weak. Diuretics, drugs that make you urinate out extra fluid, are useful in heart failure – in small, predictable doses and to a minimal degree. Commonly they were used instead for acute illnesses, like trauma or infection. Like bleeding or purgatives, they worsened a situation that was already bad. Drugs that made people sweat were used, since people believed that poisons came out of the body with sweat. They were wrong. What came out in sweat was salt and fluid – both vital for anyone already ill.

Drugs to bring on abortions or to prevent conception are old. The ancient Egyptian use of crocodile dung as a vaginal pessary actually did work – to an extent, and arguably as much by damping sexual attraction as being directly spermicidal. A very few ancient treatments actually did some good. Mercury, despite being very toxic, could help against syphilis: but not much, and often not enough to counteract its own harms. Another chemical element, antimony, has a limited ability to fight off a disease called schistosomiasis, a parasite that can be acquired from swimming in infected water in Africa. Colchicine, from the crocus, was used with some benefit to treat gout – as well as with a lot of harm to induce vomiting and diarrhoea.

Trepanation in ancient Egypt is often held up as an example of how advanced ancient surgery was. Surgeons were able to drill holes in people's skulls, to lift out pieces of bone. Skulls have been found where the wounds have healed over, showing that some people survived. The ancient Egyptians were advanced enough to sometimes remove a portion of someone's skull without killing the patient – but that does not mean they understood when doing so might be of help. They used the technique to save some of those suffering from certain types of fractured skulls. They used it to harm many whose problems were actually psychiatric, neurological or infective, and incapable of benefiting from the pain and danger of trepanation.

The inclusion of a potentially helpful ingredient in a long list of others is no indication of real knowledge or any actual healing powers. In the twentieth century, for example, knowing that something in penicillin could kill bacteria, doctors still struggled to get any practical benefits from it. With exactly the right species of mould and advanced chemical techniques to extract concentrated amounts of its juice, they still found it exceedingly difficult to make it do anything useful. Getting a therapeutic effect from the *Penicillium* fungus was that hard. This tells us something important about how to interpret the fact that some Egyptian wound dressings included mouldy bread.

So something else matters, beyond the pharmacological properties of a drug: people's ability to harness it. Were the Greeks and the Romans able to use opium to *reliably* or even *usually* bring an end to pain? Did they make operations comfortable, death easy, illnesses mild? No. Even by the nineteenth century doctors were unable to do these things, remaining too confused about doses and preparations, too uncertain of effects, and too frightened of side effects.

2 Sophistry and Laudanum

An early step forwards in the history of science came with a philosophical argument amongst the ancient Greeks. Five hundred years before the birth of Christ, a group of Greeks made their living from their skills in argument. Athens was a litigious society, and success or failure in lawsuits often depended on such skills. This group of men were called sophists, initially as a compliment to their wisdom and, later, as something of an insult to their morals. ('Sophistry' came to mean arguing for something not honestly or because it was true, but with lies and confusions and because doing so served your own selfish interests.) The sophists rejected the widespread belief that the best way to understand the world was to reason it out. They argued that experience, rather than pure reason, gave you more accurate information about the way the world actually was.

One of the greatest opponents of the sophists was Plato. His belief was that experience of the world was misleading. The ground that we walked on and the buildings and people and shapes around us were only versions – imitations – of what was most real. That deeper truth was hidden. The mind could attempt to figure out, through the power of thought, the pure forms of this underlying reality. Experience only got distracted and confused by the jumbled reflections of it. Experiments could tell you only about these illusions and superficialities, not about anything more important. Those who believed in such barbarically practical methods as experiments were called 'empirics'. It was a term of contempt.

Aristotle argued against this belief in the value of speculation. Reason had to be founded on experience, he suggested. Philosophy was not enough to tell you about how a bee managed to fly or the number of teeth in a person's head. Instead you needed to study the bee, or to open up someone's mouth and start counting what you saw. The words 'experiment' and 'experience' still meant pretty much the same to Aristotle, but at least he felt that something important was hidden away in them. It was an idea that rumbled away in the human mind, not emerging into anything that saved lives or eased pains, but packed, all the same, with promise.

Aristotle complained that Plato relied too much on his own thoughts, his own ability to reason from nothing about how the world worked. That was not, suspected Aristotle, quite good enough. Why should the world work the way you expected it to? It seemed better to him to start by observing what was around you, and then to move on to trying to think through what you saw. Fitting your thoughts to the world rather than the world to your thoughts held more promise of getting things right. Aristotle's belief was in what he called 'natural philosophy', in basing your knowledge on your experiences. Thomas Aquinas rephrased this belief seventeen centuries later: *Nihil est in intellectu quod non prius in sensu*, 'Nothing is in the intellect which was not first in the senses.' Experience, both men believed, was more reliable than innate wisdom, at least when it came to understanding the truth about the natural world.

A lot of thought and effort went into working out what it was about experience that was helpful. Certain forms of experience seemed more useful than others. Organising observations made them more reliable; the notion that *experiments* were vital grew in people's minds.

Roughly a thousand years after the birth of Christ, Ibn al-

Haytham was born in Basra, in the south of modern Iraq. His book on optics explored the nature of vision and included the most developed statement yet of scientific method. Observations, said al-Haytham, gave rise in people's minds to problems, which they then developed theories to explain. Those theories then needed experimental examination. Both al-Haytham's approach and his optical knowledge greatly impressed Roger Bacon, the thirteenth-century English philosopher friar. Bacon stressed that observation, theorising and experimentation provided the means for finding out about the reality of the world. He documented his experiments in detail, precisely so that others could repeat them and check on his results.

Bacon's emphasis on verification contained an acknowledgement of his fallibility. Never before had anyone so seriously tried to build in safeguards against their own aptitude for errors and confusions. The decline of mental arrogance, the dissolution of people's instinctive belief in the accuracy of their intuition, was ever so gradually progressing.

In the late sixteenth century the unrelated Francis Bacon helped to popularise this view of scientific method. 'Men have sought to make a world from their own conception', he wrote, 'and to draw from their own minds all the material which they employed, but if, instead of doing so, they had consulted experience and observation, they would have the facts and not opinions to reason about, and might have ultimately arrived at the knowledge of the laws which govern the material world.'

Francis Bacon (his eyes like those of a viper, according to the contemporary physician William Harvey) died in the manner of a true scientist. A winter coach-ride in the company of the king's physician, Dr Witherborne, prompted him to wonder if the snow, lying round about, might preserve meat. Consumed with curiosity, the two men plunged out of their coach and into the nearest house, persuading the woman who lived there to sell them a live chicken.

They had her kill and gut the creature, and Bacon, full of enthusiasm, grabbed handfuls of snow to help stuff it with. 'The Snow so chilled him that he immediately fell so extremely ill, that he could not returne to his Lodging,' wrote the gossipy biographer John Aubrey towards the end of the seventeenth century, some fifty years after the events he confidently recounted. '2 or 3 dayes' after, probably having been bled by his travelling companion, he died of pneumonia. Later opinion on his life was mixed. 'If parts allure thee, think how Bacon shined,' wrote Alexander Pope in the eighteenth century, 'The wisest, brightest, meanest of mankind.'

These advances in thinking about the need to experiment were important scientifically but not medically. They changed nothing about the way patients were treated. Seeing a doctor for professional advice remained a bad choice. This is not to say that doctors were universally awful, or even that they did not occasionally do good, only that their overall impact on the human race was to diminish it – to shorten lives and extend disease. Surgeons could set simple fractures and perform basic operations, often to the benefit of their patients. But without the idea of infection the wounds they created frequently went bad, and even the shallowest scratch of a doctor's needle let in the possibility of death. In the seventeenth century the Norfolk doctor Thomas Browne was greatly taken with Bacon's methods, as well as with another great find of the time: William Harvey's discovery of the circulation of the blood. 'Be sure', he wrote, 'you make yourself master of Dr Harvey's piece *De Circul. Sang.*; which discovery I prefer to that of Columbus.' After thousands of years of ignorance, Harvey showed in the seventeenth century that the heart pumped blood in a circuit around the body. It was a terrific insight, more impressive to Browne than the discovery of the Americas, but it led to not a single change in the way doctors treated their patients. It did not even prompt them to reconsider their enthusiasm for bleeding and leeches.

*

These new ways of thinking played a central part in the life of Theophrastus Phillipus Aureolus Bombastus von Hohenheim – or, as he took to calling himself, Paracelsus. He was born in Switzerland in 1493 and the name he chose signified his sense of superiority to the Roman medical authority Celsus. It was a superiority that Paracelsus declared for himself. His career took him across the known European world, searching out knowledge and its mad relations. Paracelsus took a florid interest in the theories, intuitions and products of his own genius, combining them with armfuls of the occult, of alchemy and of more straightforward natural philosophy. 'When I saw that nothing resulted from [medical] practice but killing and laming, I determined to abandon such a miserable art and seek truth elsewhere.' His low opinion of contemporary medicine was accurate. Like many of those who held it over the centuries, his consequent belief that he could do very much better was wildly off the mark.

The mental techniques with which Paracelsus armed himself were weak and treacherous. The 'doctrine of signatures', which pre-dated written histories, was one of his favourites. It held that inner powers could be determined by superficial appearances. When it came to medicine, this meant that similarities between a plant and a disease were taken to be proof of a therapeutic link. Gold cured jaundice since both were yellow, flowers that looked like testicles cured sexual diseases, the prickles of thistles mended prickly internal pains. It is an idea found in many societies, and neither its long heritage nor its attractive simplicity moves it any closer to being truthful. Other men trusted their intuitions and came up with therapies that were harmful. Paracelsus mocked them for it, then made up some of his own. More usefully, perhaps, he also equipped himself with a large sword. It was handy in itself, for a wandering and pugnacious soul in the medieval world, but within its hilt was something even better. He stuffed his sword with riches. 'I possess a secret remedy,' he declared, 'which I call laudanum and which is superior to all other heroic remedies.'

This pioneer of a new medicine talked a good revolution. 'If I want to prove anything,' he said, 'I shall not do so by quoting authorities but by experiment and by reasoning thereupon. I do not believe in the ancient doctrine of complexions and humours which has been falsely supposed to account for all diseases. It is because of these doctrines that so few physicians have correct views of disease, its origins and its course.' His 'experiments', however, were extensions of his own faith and intuition, their results folded up into theories so curdled and capacious that they contained all possible outcomes. Paracelsus talked like a scientist but his 'truths' were often fabulously complex delusions. He used the scientific jargon of the day, adopted the words and the traditions of emerging chemistry, and applied them in a manner as misleading as that of the mistaken Greeks, Romans and Arabs he viciously scorned. 'I tell you, one hair on my neck knows more than all you authors, and my shoe-buckles contain more wisdom than both Galen and Avicenna.' So much for his boasts. What, however, was this laudanum in the pommel of his sword?

The miracle cure that Paracelsus carried around with him certainly looked strange. It consisted of what he called 'Stones of Immortality', which looked a bit like the droppings of an odd and furtive animal. Citrus juice, gold and other more unlikely ingredients were combined with opium. In fact, the only part of them that had a real effect was the opium. And it was an effect that people rather liked.

They liked it not least because it really could increase their chances of living. So long as doctors like Paracelsus believed that it could cure them, they set aside their more dangerous alternative remedies. And while laudanum, like any form of opium, could be dangerous in overdose, compared to the rest of what the doctors used it was often safer than water.

What Paracelsus discovered was a more potent form of opium, a way of concentrating it. He dissolved the poppy's dried latex in alcohol rather than water. That added an extra dose of spirits to the medicine itself. It also meant, since the active compounds within the poppy dissolved far more easily in alcohol, that the pharmacological kick per pint was considerably greater.

Paracelsus died in 1541. Eighty-three years later, in the summer of 1624, a baby was born in the English county of Dorset. Thomas Sydenham grew up in a world whose medicine as well as its school teaching remained heavily Greek and Roman. Subsequent advances in anatomy and in scientific method continued to be of little use to those who sought help from physicians, apothecaries or surgeons. Still, with an Oxford education and much natural sense (the more useful of the two, given the quality of England's universities at the time), Sydenham was able to recognise a good thing. The poppy impressed him. He declared that 'among the remedies which it has pleased the Almighty God to give to man to relieve his sufferings, none is so universal and so efficacious as opium'.

Not that anyone yet understood how opium worked. Molière's mockery in *Le Malade imaginaire* of 1673 made fun of the pompous jargon with which doctors hid their ignorance.

'I have been asked by a learned doctor what is the cause and reason why opium induces sleep,' says a medical student, hoping to be granted a licence to practise as a fully qualified doctor. 'To which I reply it is because there is in it a dormitive virtue, the nature of which is to sedate the senses.' His examiners are delighted with his excellent response.

Thomas Sydenham's commitment to fresher ways of looking at the world bit deep into his life. His first session of study at Oxford

ended when the Civil War broke out in 1642, and Sydenham went off
to fight for the cause of Parliament and democracy against the
Divine Right of the kings. He returned, having lost two brothers and
a great quantity of his own blood, and finished his studies. But, he
wrote, 'I became convinced that the physician who earnestly studies,
with his own eyes – and not through the medium of books . . . must
necessarily excel.' His Oxford education was entirely based on
books; for a physician to study anything else was seen as being
beneath such highly qualified men. Sydenham believed otherwise,
and did his best to persuade others. A junior colleague asked for
advice about the most useful books to study. 'Read *Don Quixote*,' he
was told, '. . . a very good book; I read it still.' It was not only the
uselessness of contemporary textbooks that he was highlighting, but
his own reputation for Quixotic eccentricity. It seemed more than a
little mad for a doctor not to put his whole faith in the teaching of his
elders.

Robert Boyle, the Royal Society chemist, described Sydenham to
a mutual friend as a 'ripe scholar, a good botanist, and a skilled
anatomist'. The friend repeated the praise, only for Sydenham to
surprise him by responding:

This is all very fine, but it won't do – Anatomy – Botany –
Nonsense! Sir, I know an old woman in Covent Garden who
understands botany better, and as for anatomy, my butcher can
dissect a joint full and well; no, young man, all that is stuff; you
must go to the bedside, it is there alone you can learn disease.

His frank views went along with enough personal warmth to
make him attractive to many leading thinkers. Boyle was a close
friend, as was the philosopher Locke. Yet for all Sydenham's
advances in epistemology and observation, for all that he prompted
doctors to pay more attention to the natural history of diseases,

recording their signs and symptoms, progressions and outcomes, the benefit for patients was almost nil. In the end, Sydenham's greatest therapeutic tool was his willingness to withhold medicines. 'The arrival of a good clown exercises a more beneficial influence upon the health of a town', he wrote, 'than of twenty asses laden with drugs.' Finding a patient brought to a state of physical and emotional collapse – not by disease, but by the drugs that others had given to bring on vomiting and diarrhoea – Sydenham 'therefore ordered him a roast chicken and a pint of canary'.

Sydenham's therapeutic nihilism, a disbelief in the purported value of medicines, was profound. 'I confidently affirm that the greater part of those who are supposed to have died of gout', Sydenham declared, 'have died of the medicine rather than the disease.' As a gout sufferer himself, he worked his way through the available treatments, concluding that they were more toxic than therapeutic. He was not the first to decide that masterly inactivity was frequently the best option, but he was unusually open in his views. 'It is a great mistake to suppose that Nature always stands in need of the assistance of Art,' he argued, referring to the art of a doctor. 'I have consulted the safety of my patient and my own reputation effectually by doing nothing at all.'

Sydenham's approach to bleeding verged on the revolutionary – rather than calling for a leech or a lancet at every opportunity, he called for them with relative moderation. He recognised the benefits of laudanum, although he was not able to distinguish between those of the drug itself and those it brought about by helping a patient to escape from more poisonous 'cures'. He was suspicious of the extra ingredients added by Paracelsus, and simplified the recipe. In a medical world that prized the complexity of drugs – the more stuff, and the more exotic, the better – this was an accurate and fairly original intuition. Woodlice, human skulls, supposed unicorn horn, pearls, snakes and the contents of animal guts were routinely added to preparations. It was called polypharmacy, indicating the number of constituents, and it carried on until nineteenth-century chemists became confident that what was important were the properties of particular active ingredients – an insight that developed into the idea of molecular receptors, cellular locks that responded only to keys of a specific microscopic structure.

For laudanum, Sydenham recommended two parts of opium to one of saffron, along with some cinnamon and some cloves, all mixed in with sweet wine. Cloves possess some mild local anaesthetic properties, but like the other spice and the choice of a popular (and relatively expensive) drink, their main purpose was far more practical. They tasted good. That helped the medicine go down. 'The act is all,' said Goethe in *Faust*, 'the reputation nothing.' Doctors knew better.

The fact that Sydenham dissolved opium in wine – canary wine, similar to the Madeira we have today – has an aspect to it that is easy to overlook. Wine and poppies went together. They provided both ease and forgetfulness and also alertness and a sharpening of the senses. When Samuel Taylor Coleridge, in 1817, wanted a word to describe what laudanum did, he coined a new one: *intensify*.

Part of the reason for our modern horror of opiates comes as a side effect of our war on drugs. The penalty for transporting coca leaves is the same as for cocaine; highly concentrated morphine the same as for the unprocessed latex of *Papaver somniferum*. Potency therefore carries a premium. If you are going to risk yourself in producing and moving illegal drugs, it is in your interests to shift them in as concentrated a form as possible. So the legal dangers of drug dealers become the physiological ones of their customers. Heroin now finds its way into every city, while the milder alternatives that were so common throughout human history – poppy tea, or home-made laudanum – have gone. All that has remained is a love of the poppy for the sake of its appearance.

How was it that doctors persisted in prescribing remedies that helped to kill their patients, yet the profession of medicine continued? How did doctors maintain a reputation for being helpful while causing harm?

The nineteenth-century Boston physician Oliver Wendell Holmes thought he had the answer. What people desired most was something to believe in, and they were willing to pay heavily for it:

> There is nothing people will not do, there is nothing they have not done, to recover their health and save their lives. They have submitted to be half drowned in water, half cooked with gasses, to be buried up to their chins in the earth, to be seared with hot irons like slaves, to be crimped with knives like codfish, to have needles thrust into their flesh, and bonfires kindled on their skin, to swallow all sorts of abomination, and to pay for all of this, as if to be singed and scaled were a costly privilege, as if blisters were a blessing and leeches were a luxury.

To this day, little in medicine is so difficult as doing nothing at all. Medicine is founded on the desire of patients to be helped and of doctors to help. These desires outweigh sense. The difficulty of doing nothing, or of admitting that there is nothing to be done, is overwhelming. Like politicians who need to be seen to be doing something – anything – about problems that are actually beyond their control, doctors are pushed into playing a part. The danger, with both doctors and politicians, comes when they start to believe in their own illusory importance. People want doctors who are confident, certain, able to offer *treatment*. The confidence that makes people trust doctors has a way of working its way into the doctor's character. Persuading people to trust your judgement is essential – if people are going to feel cared for, if they are going to feel safe enough to follow your advice, or at least to be soothed by it – and it is always easiest to persuade people if you have convinced yourself first of all.

'As for a radical cure, one altogether perfect,' wrote Sydenham, 'and one whereby a patient might be freed from even the disposition to the disease. This lies, like Truth, at the bottom of a well; and so deep is it in the innermost recesses of Nature, that I know not when or by whom it will be brought forward into the light of day.' This is good advice, but not the sort of advice a frightened patient wants to hear. The patient wants someone offering confidence and hope, not the audacity of doubt.

Francis Bacon, and the others after him who developed what we now call scientific method, were not developing ways of using pipettes, or rules about wearing white coats and working in laboratories. The mental tools they developed had nothing to do with particular pieces of laboratory equipment. Journalists talk of 'scientists' as though they are a different species from the rest of us, rather than being any person trying to make his or her beliefs more accurate by testing them. A child skimming rocks on the surface of a pond is engaged in a sort of science, gradually experimenting with the shapes of the stones and the angle of their throw to get as many bounces as possible. A man with a beard and a PhD working with sophisticated machines is, if he is not testing his theories, engaged in something that is not science at all.

Struggling to understand the best ways for learning about the world, Francis Bacon tried to work out why it was that we so often got it wrong, taking mental routes that led us away from reality. At the end of the sixteenth century and the start of the seventeenth, in small uncertain steps, he was distinguishing fertile thought from a different kind of mental activity, one that produced illusions that seemed real and mistakes that felt right. Bacon's love for truth was real to him, as was his fear of those things in his mind that distracted him from recognising it:

> The idols and false notions which are now in possession of the human understanding, and have taken deep root therein, not only so beset men's minds that truth can hardly find entrance, but even after entrance is obtained, they will again . . . meet and trouble us, unless men being forewarned of the danger fortify themselves as far as may be against their assaults.

Our minds, said Bacon, have a habit of seeing order where none exists, of making connections because they appeal to us rather than because there is evidence for them. We have individual prejudices, clouding our minds and pushing us away from the truth purely because some conclusions taste better to us than others. Words matter also, and we get some things wrong simply because we are muddled over expressing them, allowing vagueness or confusion to spill into our thoughts from the phrases we house them in. Then there are the errors brought on by success, by teachings and arguments whose popularity and appeal are beyond their actual value. Arguments are not necessarily won by those in possession of the truth, but by those who are the most persuasive.

These mental errors, Bacon said,

> have their foundation in human nature itself, and in the tribe or race of men. For it is a false assertion that the sense of man is the measure of things. On the contrary, all perceptions, as well of the sense as of the mind, are according to the measure of the individual and not according to the measure of the universe. And the human understanding is like a false mirror, which, receiving rays irregularly, distorts and discolours the nature of things by mingling its own nature with it.

Science provided a system whereby people could rescue themselves from muddles, and guard against mistakes. There was no perfect way of avoiding mental errors, any more than disease. The best that could be hoped for was to remain aware of how inevitably mistakes arose, and to use tests and trials to continually weed them out.

3 Self-confidence and Quinine

'I die by the help of too many physicians' was supposed to have been the final sentiment on the lips of Alexander the Great in 323 BC. Four hundred years later, Pliny suggested a new epitaph was becoming common, echoing Alexander. 'It was the crowd of physicians that killed me' was an easy enough sentiment for someone to declare upon his death, a harder one to accept in the days leading up to it. Blaming doctors for their failures did not stop people flocking to them hoping for success.

The knowledge that medicines were toxic was widespread, but this augmented rather than undermined the impression that doctors commanded therapeutic power. If medicines were dangerous, that meant they were powerful – and even if the power to harm was what was seen, the power to help was imagined to accompany it. It was difficult, in affliction, to resist the comforting idea of medical help. The greatest of doctors achieved their stature partly by unflinching self-belief. Galen's confidence, for example, was part of his appeal. It was confidence robust enough to survive any collision with reality. He said of one potion:

> All who drink of this treatment recover in a short time, except those whom it does not help, who all die. It is obvious, therefore, that it fails only in incurable cases.

Fevers, Galen believed, arose from an excess of blood. The treatment was therefore clear. (Galen's faith in bleeding was extreme. He even recommended it as a cure for blood loss.) For a fever, a patient should be bled twice a day, the second time to the point where they fainted. Galen based his beliefs about the human body on complex theories of internal humours and their differing effects. He was contemptuous of those healers whose lack of theoretical beliefs left them reliant on experimenting.

Bleeding stuck with phenomenal longevity in the mind of medics. Here is Sir William Osler, a founding professor at Johns Hopkins University and later the Regius Professor of Medicine at Oxford, on pneumonia:

> To bleed at the very onset in robust, healthy individuals in whom the disease sets in with great intensity and high fever is good practice.

He was writing in 1920, almost two millennia after Galen. The theories underlying the treatment had changed. Osler knew more about the human body and the microbes that cause pneumonia than Galen. What was unaltered was the effect of bleeding on a patient suffering from this infection of the lungs. It remained bad. The theories changed, the harm remained the same. Galen's poisoned gift to his profession, even more than his belief in bleeding or his list of 473 different drugs, was his complacency. He wrote:

> I have done as much for medicine as Trajan did for the Roman Empire when he built bridges and roads through Italy. It is I, and I alone, who have revealed the true path of medicine. It must be admitted that Hippocrates already staked out this path . . . he prepared the way, but I have made it passable.

One of the key infections that Galen dealt with was malaria. The characteristic cycle of chills and fevers makes descriptions of the disease by early doctors recognisable, even when they understood little of what they were recording. Malaria is caused by a protozoan parasite, a single-celled organism with a cell wall and a means of propulsion – the latter making it a little more like an animal than a plant. *Plasmodium*, the protozoan genus concerned, has infected humans long enough for many of us to have evolved genetic defences to it. Most likely it has existed as long as our species, since related protozoans affect chimps and other primates. It seems to have originated, like us, in Africa. When people migrated, they took it with them. The *plasmodium* spends only part of its life in humans, taking up residence the rest of the time in mosquitoes. The bite of a mosquito is the way in which the disease spreads from person to person – or, to put it from the insect's point of view, malaria goes from one mosquito to another when they eat from the same walking table.

For the First World, malaria today is a holiday problem. Elsewhere, two thirds of a billion people fall sick with it each year and several million, mostly African children, die. There are no vaccines. Drugs, however, can successfully protect against and treat the disease. The oldest of these is the bark of a South American tree, cinchona, containing a compound called quinine which is poisonous to the protozoan.

In England the disease used to be called the ague, from a word for fever. It came upon people for no obvious reason, although many linked it to swamps and to foul air. Not until Horace Walpole fled Rome in the summer of 1740, keen to escape the disease, did the English begin to adopt their modern term. There is, said Walpole, writing home to a friend, 'a horrid thing called the mal'aria, that comes to Rome every summer and kills one, and I did not care for being killed so far from Christian burial'.

The swamps and marshes around Rome, as Walpole observed, were known to give rise to the disease. Religion, at least as judged by one's rank in the Church, was no defence: popes and cardinals lived in fear of malaria, and died as easily as their humbler brethren.

Around 150 years before Walpole's letter, at the start of the seventeenth century, the Spanish had begun bringing back to Europe the bark of a particular South American tree. Jesuit priests in Peru found that the natives used it, chiefly for treating wounds. The *quina-quina* tree gave out a balsam, and as well as being useful for wounds it seemed to work for fevers. It had no particular value for malaria, but its use caught on all the same. This 'Peruvian balsam bark', however, was expensive. To supply the demand, merchants began sending home an alternative bark instead. At first it was used haphazardly and without great interest. The prevailing atmosphere was hostile to innovation: in 1624 Pope Urban VIII issued a papal bull excommunicating all smokers of the newly introduced tobacco; in 1633 he demanded that Galileo recant his ideas about the universe.

Others were more open to new ideas. In 1643 a Belgian doctor referred to the substitute bark – which came to be called *árbol de calenturas* or fever tree – being used in Europe to treat malarial fevers. It also took the name quinine, from the original *quina-quina* tree that it had been introduced to replace. Interest in Rome was driven by Juan de Lugo, a Spanish cardinal, who kept a supply of the bark, selling it at great price to the rich and giving it away freely to the poor. This bark, ground into powder, was the first European medicine that actually cured the patients who took it. Opiates dulled pain, but did not increase survival. For the first time in history, here was a drug that did something better. It was miraculous, and yet faith in existing nostrums was so profound that most people failed to notice.*

* A parallel can be made with anatomy. The teachings of Galen, which had muddled up human and non-human anatomical structures, overpowered the early anatomists. When, in the dawning Renaissance, they began to open up human corpses and look with their own eyes, their prejudices misled them. Even men like Leonardo da Vinci saw and drew not what was in front of them, but what Galen had taught them to expect. Their expectations moulded their experience. It is hard to imagine a clearer example of the fallibilities of human insight and observation.

When Urban VIII died in 1644, fear of the Roman malaria meant many cardinals refused to cross the fever-ridden flatlands surrounding the city for the conclave picking his successor. In the year that Innocent X was elected to his office, Cardinal de Lugo asked the new Pope's doctor what he thought of the powder's power. The verdict was glowing, although the papal physician saw nothing out of the ordinary about the powder's excellence. In the next few years Juan de Lugo's reputation and influence rose. He began distributing the bark more widely, both from his own house and from the Collegio Romano, the supreme seminary of the Jesuits. It was taken up more enthusiastically for being patronised by this powerful base. Major Jesuit congregations were held in Rome in the years 1646, 1649 and 1650. Desire for the *pulvis cardinalis* or *pulvis Jesuiticus* – the cardinal's powder, the Jesuits powder – grew. De Lugo, supported by Innocent X, preached to the Jesuits of its utility. The impressed brethren returned to their corners of the Catholic empire with enthusiasm on their lips.

By 1651 the powder had found its way onto an official formulary, a list of permissible and recognised drugs. The *Schedula Romana*, amongst the hundreds of useless and harmful medications, now included one that healed. The next year, 1652, Archduke Leopold of Austria was struck down with a malarial fever. Treated with the new bark, as recommended in the *Schedula Romana*, Leopold rapidly recovered. A month later, however, he became feverish again. Rather than opting for another dose of the excellent powder, Leopold 'was so incensed that . . . he ordered his physician to write a book attacking the remedy and warning against its dangers'. Other doctors joined in, their own prejudices trumping their ability to perceive the drug's life-saving effects. In 1655, bubonic plague hit Rome, and when the feverish victims of this quite different disease were treated with Jesuits' powder they got no better. The bark fell out of favour.

*

In south-east England the marshes were as deadly as those of the Roman flatlands. *Anopheles atroparvus* was the mosquito that spread English malaria, and parish records showed that it harvested a great many souls. For hundreds of years the death rates in marshland parishes were greater than births – only a constant influx of migrants kept the communities from slipping whole into their sodden graves. The country was ripe for the arrival of an effective treatment against malaria. The Jesuit bark, however, was too much of a Catholic invention to be trusted by such a Protestant country.

One man with no qualms about Catholicism, orthodoxy or innovation was Kenelm Digby. When Kenelm was a toddler his Catholic father Everard tried to blow up the Houses of Parliament. Along with Guy Fawkes and the other plotters he went to the scaffold.* Kenelm lived a life of romance, piracy, politics and science. When his wife died in 1633 he was heartbroken, commissioning a eulogy by Ben Jonson and a portrait by Van Dyck before retreating for comfort to his academic researches. He played a part in discovering oxygen, authored a famous cookbook (*The Closet of the Eminently Learned Sir Kenelme Digbie Knight Opened*, published posthumously in 1669), helped found the Royal Society and developed the modern form of the wine bottle (strengthening the glass so that the wine inside could slowly mature). He also popularised his 'Powder of Sympathy'. Crossing the line between natural philosophy and magic – a line whose location was as unclear to Digby as to his contemporary Newton – this was a preparation of copper sulphate believed to harness astrological powers. It was to treat wounds, but not to be applied to them. Instead the powder was meant to go on the weapon that had caused them. 'Sympathy' would cause the wound to heal in response. In a real way it was a genuine life-saver – in a world where poultices

---

* John Aubrey reported the death. The executioner, he said, pulled out Everard's heart and announced it to be that of a traitor. 'Thou liest!' replied the dying man.

and dressings were toxic and infested with germs, slapping a treatment on a weapon rather than a wound was, a great protection to the suffering.

Having fled England during the early 1640s, and stayed away during the Civil War, Kenelm Digby returned in 1655. He brought with him news of 'the bark of a tree that infallibly cureth all intermittent fevers. It cometh from Peru, and is that bark of a tree called by the Spaniards kina-kina.' (Confusion over exactly what tree the bark really came from persisted, problematically. Contemporary reports muddle up the Peruvian balsam tree with the cinchona that produced quinine. To add to the chaos there were also many different types of cinchona, some of which contained so little of the key drug as to be useless.)

Three years later, in 1658, the treatment using cinchona – what Digby called kina-kina – was being advertised in the English press, a London weekly newspaper carrying a notice that 'the excellent powder, known by the name of "Jesuits' Powder", may be obtained . . . at the lodgings of Mr James Thompson, merchant from Antwerp, or at Mr John Crook's, bookseller, with directions for its use'.

Despite the swell of popular interest, and even the approval of the president of the Royal College of Physicians, no one was really certain what to make of the powder. That year an alderman of the City of London was given it. He died. In a country where Catholics were blamed for everything, the Jesuitical powder was suspected of being murderous. When Oliver Cromwell fell ill with malaria that September, it was said that he refused to touch a powder so tainted with papacy, submitting instead to the treatments of his physicians, whose bleedings and drugs helped hurry him into the grave.*

*

* The branding of a drug, even in the seventeenth century, was everything. The story of Cromwell refusing the powder was apocryphal. The prejudice against the powder was real.

Robert Talbor grew up in the marshy fens of Cambridgeshire. He attended the university there for a few years but left in 1668 without getting a degree. He chose to settle in Essex. The coastal swamps of the county appealed to him, he said, for exactly the reasons other people might want to avoid them. 'I planted myself near the seaside,' explained Tabor, 'where the agues are the epidemical diseases.'

Four years later he was confident enough in his researches to publish them. Going into print was a fine way then, as it is today, for a doctor to attract a reputation and a paying clientele. Talbor warned people away from Jesuits' powder, 'for I have seen most dangerous effects follow the taking of the Medicine'. He did admit that in the right hands this 'Powder [was] not altogether to be condemned' but said he had something better to offer, something less tainted by associations with Rome.

The early history of Talbor's efforts was partially uncovered when Rudolph Siegel, a twentieth-century medical historian researching Galen and his teachings, bought a copy of Leclerc's 1702 *Histoire de la médecine*. There, scribbled on the fly-leaves, was a first-hand account of 'how Quinquina became finally established all over Europe'. Siegel and a colleague were unable to determine the name of the man who wrote it, but established that he was a French nobleman. From 1672 to 1678 France and the Dutch were at war, and for two years from 1672 England joined in on the side of the French. The unidentified French nobleman was recuperating at that time in England. 'Being very ill with an intermittent fever which I contracted in Flanders and which afflicted almost our entire army during that year, the woman attending our quarters brought to me a very poor man who had cured several of my servants.' The man was Robert Talbor and, despite his appearance of dishevelled poverty, his self-confidence was enough for the French officer to swallow the cure that he offered, 'a powder steeped in a large glass of white wine'. It worked:

I was able to embark on my week's service at the Court of King Charles II, who however had to go by water to Sheerness, the most fever-ridden place in the whole of England. I told this to my little doctor, who gave me permission not only to go there, but also to amuse myself swimming, and even in debauchery if I felt inclined. Thus, when I went on board ship I could not avoid telling the whole story to the most inquisitive King in the whole world, who is also the greatest patron of empirics.

The description of Charles II's interest in and support for science was accurate. On 28 November 1660, only a few months after his Restoration, the Society of London for the Improvement of Natural Knowledge was founded. Known as the Royal Society, it was supported by the monarch who gave it its charter in 1662. Fighting against the pervasive influence of dogma – of inherited wisdom – the Society sought to pursue new ways of finding out about the world. Knowledge was no longer to be something that belonged to people by virtue of their eminence and reputation; instead it was for all those who knew the methods for finding it. This was Francis Bacon's 'experimental' philosophy. The Society's motto, *Nullius in Verba*, may be roughly translated as 'Nothing in Words'. No matter how respected or senior a teacher, what he said was not to be taken as dogma. Members of the Royal Society wanted conclusions that followed unavoidably from clearly described and repeatable experiments, not the words of experts. Like Talbor, the Royal Society was interested in quinine and performed experiments with it. Despite Bacon's efforts however, the Society's broader idea – that truth was something that needed to be uncovered by rigorous experiment – remained radical.

The ingredients of Talbor's medicine were his secret. He wrote that it consisted of 'a preparation of four vegetables', two being

45

foreign and two domestic. Hearing about its powers, Charles II demanded to meet Talbor, and, according to the French nobleman, personally organised experiments. He asked his own physicians to analyse Tabor's cure, to see what it contained that had so powerful an effect. When they proved unable to do this, the king 'gave [Talbor] a pension of 300 pieces and a Knighthood and made him one of his personal physicians'. The deal was that Talbor would reveal his ingredients to the king, and in return the king would keep the secret safe for the length of Talbor's life. The secret turned out, of course, to be Jesuit bark, fashionably repackaged. (The other 'vegetables' were rose leaves, lemon juice and, mixing everything together, grapes in the form of wine.)

Charles II used Talbor's success to poke fun at his physicians. Following the death of the London alderman from the Jesuit bark, they 'had expressly forbidden . . . Quinquina as a useless and dangerous drug'. Then, in 1679 while at Windsor Palace, Charles II fell ill with malaria. Convinced that Jesuit bark was the only thing that could save his life, he demanded to be given it. His royal wish was granted, and he rapidly recovered. 'After which, the King . . . pressed Dr. Lower maliciously, asking him how the very thing which was so bad for [him] had become so wonderfully good for him.'

Embarrassed, Dr Lower replied 'that this was a remedy from which only kings were worthy of profiting'. It was as close as the royal physician could get to admitting an error.

Other accounts hold that it was with Louis XIV that Talbor struck his deal for a pension and secrecy, in return for the ingredients and the right to publish them for the benefits of mankind after Talbor's death. Certainly it is true that, once Talbor died in 1681, *The English Remedy or Talbor's Wonderful Secret for Curing of Agues and Fevers*, was published originally in French and by Louis's own doctor.* The account of Talbor's dealings with Charles II, however, were noted down at first hand by the French nobleman who introduced them.

Whatever the truth of the slightly conflicting details, two things are certain. Jesuits' bark slowly became established as an effective remedy – although its popularity, despite the fact it was unique as a curative therapy, neither exceeded nor replaced that for bleeding. (Even by the middle of the nineteenth century, bleeding, vomiting and drugs to cause diarrhoea were, along with 'the unlimited use of coffee and whisky . . . the treatments for malaria favoured particularly by the [American] frontiersmen'.) Secondly, the world had changed in other ways. Curiosity and empiricism were becoming respectable.

Cinchona – Jesuits' Bark – is not an example of the tremendous wisdom of traditional therapies. It is difficult to know how it was originally used amongst the natives of South America, but it was not for malaria. Until the Europeans arrived and inadvertently brought it with them, that disease did not exist.

What seems to have been discovered early on by the South Americans, before malaria arrived, was that certain barks reduced fevers. To the extent that they used bark to ease symptoms and suffering, they were using it in a way that deserves the name of medicine. Fever, though, is not a disease. Instead it is part of the body's response to infection, part of the body's defence against illness. Living creatures, even very simple ones, are exquisitely sensitive to temperature. When we are infected, our bodies raise their core temperatures purposefully. This makes us uncomfortable, distressed, even delirious and confused, but it makes life more difficult for invading infective organisms. We suffer when our core temperature rises, but bacteria breeding within us suffer more.

* Talbor definitely went to France. In 1677, when her own doctors were attempting to cure Louis's niece of malaria by making her vomit to the point of collapse, Talbor was there with his alternative remedy.

Reducing an adult's fever, in other words, can have two sorts of effect. It can make you feel better. And, by stopping your body fighting off an infection, it can make you actually get sicker. Abolishing a fever can be like going into battle with your eyes shut: the experience might cause less distress, but you are not necessarily safer.

Cinchona for malaria acts differently. The South Americans and the Europeans that started using it did so because they thought it reduced fever – which it does. But it also directly kills the *plasmodium* that causes malaria. The fever fades away partly because the drug directly reduces it, but also subsides because the drug kills the living creature that prompts the fever to begin with.

On 30 July 1809, the British landed in the Low Countries, in what is now Holland. Their force of almost 40,000 troops was the largest of their long campaign against the armies of Napoleon's France. Their aim was to destroy a major French fleet (which had already moved somewhere else) and to support the Austrians (who had already been defeated).

The British occupied a swamp-filled island called Walcheren. During the four and a half months they spent there, over 4,000 of their men died. Just over a hundred lost their lives in battle; the rest succumbed to feverish illness. Malaria, possibly in combination with typhus, was chiefly responsible. The British withdrew in December. More than a year later 12,000 campaign veterans were still sick.

The military need for Jesuit bark was clear. Yet getting hold of the bark was not easy. The cinchonas grew thousands of metres above sea level in spectacularly inaccessible regions of the Andes, protected by the Amazon to one side and the rainforest to the other. Added to this the trees varied hugely in hue, shape and size, and they hybridised with one another so cheerfully as to be perpetually incon-sistent to those who wanted to harvest them.

48

In the wake of Vesalius's 1543 *De humani corporis fabrica*, anatomy had come to be studied seriously and methodically. The long eighteenth century had seen widespread developments in physiology, while chemistry had developed into a discipline that was beginning to correctly identify elements and compounds. In the second decade of the nineteenth century – too late for the soldiers of Walcheren – several people successfully isolated the most active compound within cinchona bark. Quinine, as it came to be called, was found at different concentrations in the different species of trees. Pelletier and Caventou published their 1820 'Chemical Researches on the Quinquinas' in the Parisian scientific journal *Annales de Chimie et de Physique*. The paper opened up the way to identifying the most useful varieties of cinchona, but otherwise the discovery was strictly an advance in *Chimie* and not in *Physique*. Identifying the active ingredient of cinchona did not enable anyone to manufacture it. The molecules of living organisms were not only beyond the reach of chemists, they were thought to be permanently so. These 'organic' molecules, as they were called, were believed only to result from the processes of living cells, not from the experiments of chemists. Many believed that this was because they contained some fragment of soul, some portion of a quality that had been placed there by God in His creation of life. Human efforts to do the same with artifice were widely held to be futile.

Unable to manufacture quinine themselves, people continued their efforts to get hold of the tree. From 1829, European attempts to remove cinchona seeds from South America for cultivation elsewhere in their empires were supplemented by plans to steal away entire trees. Nathaniel Ward, a British family doctor from London, while attempting to devise better ways of hatching out butterflies, discovered a way of protecting living plants in sealed boxes. These Wardian cases made transportation easier, enabling the importation of exotic flowers and the successful smuggling of precious tea plants out of China. The cinchona proved more difficult. From the late 1850s a host of repeated efforts were under way, with English explorers like Richard Spruce, Clements Markham and Charles Ledger organising expeditions to find, transport and replant seeds and seedlings.

Success came only gradually. International cultivation of cinchona proceeded energetically as the nineteenth century closed, but early results were mixed. Initial plantings abroad were in the Dutch colony of Java and the English ones of India and what was then Ceylon. Only in the twentieth century did these efforts, combined with the over-exploitation of natural sources in South America, lead to the bulk of quinine coming from cultivation.

Medical recognition that quinine was effective for treating malaria was largely a matter of luck. The treatment was so good that haphazard observations were sufficient to notice it. It meant that doctors were more effective than they had been before, but no better able to understand the means by which they could continue to improve. What was missing was method.

4   Learning to Experiment

The Sumerians smeared their wounds with salves. Acids and herbs were some of the ingredients, others were salt, oil, juniper berries, beer, wine, mud and animal fat. Some of these, like salt and strong acids or alkalis, are quite capable of killing bacteria – but kill human cells as well. Others, like mud and meat, contain the sort of germs you want to keep as far away from damaged flesh as possible. Yet intervention remained easier for people to believe in than leaving well alone. After the civilisation of Sumer faded, the Egyptians were covering up their own wounds with similar mixes of meat, grease, honey, ostrich eggs, figs, milk, antelope fat and willow leaves.

What was lacking was not so much a drug that would kill infections – or even a comprehensive understanding of what infections actually were – but a way of being able to tell what worked from what did not. People believed in their own instincts, in the reliability of their intuitions.

They were wrong. Many wounds got better by themselves, many healed up despite being covered with muck. Others festered and people died. Yet without structure to their observations, it was impossible to reliably distinguish the effects of luck from those of useful treatments. Cinchona, when it arrived, had a tremendous effect on malaria, yet people were still opting for bleeding – which helped kill – three hundred years after cinchona reached Europe.

What chance did anyone have of noticing a drug whose effect was not massive, like cinchona's, but only moderate?

Ninth-century Baghdad was the world's most cultured city, as well as the largest. Greek medical texts were translated into Arabic, sponsoring both a reverence for ancient knowledge and a fresh interest in adding to it. Abu Bakr Muhammad ibn Zakariyya al-Razi, otherwise known as Rhazes, began studying medicine seriously only in his thirties, around the end of the century. He describes one of the first very deliberate comparisons of two alternative treatments among a group of similar patients:

> When the dullness and the pain in the head and neck continue for three and four and five days or more, and the vision shuns light, and watering of the eyes is abundant, yawning and stretching are great, insomnia is severe, and extreme exhaustion occurs, then the patient after that will progress to meningitis . . . So when you see these symptoms, then proceed with bloodletting. For I once saved one group by it, while I intentionally neglected another group. By doing that, I wished to reach a conclusion. And so all of these contracted meningitis.

Confusingly, Rhazes is describing a group of patients who already exhibit the symptoms of meningitis. With the covering of their central nervous system inflamed, they cannot move their necks without painfully stretching their spinal cord. The light hurts their retina, the exposed (and now sensitive) portion of brain at the back of the eye. They are affected so badly that their consciousness has been clouded, the yawning and the stretching replacing the brain's normal functioning. Rhazes is talking about a group of critically sick patients: the ones that he bleeds recover, the others do not.

Methodologically, he has made a step that verges on being brilliant. Dividing patients up into two identical groups, then testing one strategy on some and a different one on the others, is exactly the way of telling the difference between the effects of luck and a treatment. Yet Rhazes reaches the wrong conclusion. Meningitis is a swelling of the meninges, the membrane covering the brain and spinal cord. Bacteria and viruses can cause meningitis, as can tuberculosis and trauma. Nothing that causes meningitis benefits from blood-letting.

Rhazes does not describe how he chooses to divide his patients up. Since he was a prominent translator of Galen, we know that Rhazes's belief in blood-letting was profound. Were the patients he 'intentionally neglected' already sicker to start with, less promising for someone who wanted to show that blood-letting worked? Did he look after those whom he bled more carefully, or did they themselves feel encouraged by the treatment? How many patients were in the two groups? Given that some people with meningitis recover, and some die, were there enough to make sure that a run of luck did not distort his results?

Rhazes not only reached the wrong conclusion, he was also not particularly taken with his methods. The promise of his technique did not strike him as anything special. If it had contradicted his prejudice, and showed that those who were *not* bled did best, perhaps it might have pricked him into taking more notice. Rhazes showed some understanding of the power of comparisons, but in such a clumsy way as to make his example useless. We can see it as a flicker of mental development, a glimpse of something that could change the world – but not yet the real thing.

Rhazes had studied medicine in Baghdad, but he was born in Rayy, an ancient city that once dominated nearby Tehran and has now been absorbed within it. A generation later, another doctor from Rayy was innovating again, pursuing the idea that knowledge must be approached in a methodical way. Ibn Hindu (Abu al-Faraj Ali ibn al-Husayn) wrote that a doctor could gain knowledge in a number of ways. It could come as an accident, a natural experiment, something that you only needed to pay attention to in order to profit from. He gave the example of a boy who ate a laurel seed and then, being bitten by a snake, did not suffer. He felt that this was enough to demonstrate the protective properties of the seed. Alternatively, knowledge could be sought quite deliberately, 'by making experiments with a purpose in mind'. You could do this by 'trying several medicines one by one on bodies with different natures, time after time'. He did this himself, establishing to his own satisfaction that a plant known for causing diarrhoea could get rid of an excess of yellow bile, while another similar one got rid of black bile.

The problem was that his philosophy went nowhere. He was right that nature sometimes threw up circumstances which could teach you things, but wrong in his presumption that he could differentiate them from coincidences. Eating a laurel seed does not protect you from snake bite. Equally the idea of repeatedly trialling a drug until you could see what it did was a good one, but Ibn Hindu did not know how to do it. Both of the plants he talked of were perfectly good at causing diarrhoea, but the notion that they got rid of black or yellow bile – even the idea that the body actually contained these things in the way he imagined – was mistaken.

Ibn Hindu stressed the need for aspiring physicians to begin their studies with a thorough training in logic. It did not prevent his being unable to distinguish coincidence from causality, or from experimenting in such a crude way that he saw what he wished to see rather than what was actually occurring. Without the right methods even the most intelligent and well-meaning of scholars could be misled.

In the same century, other efforts to think about the proper way of testing treatments brought similar same mistakes. The first government-sponsored index of medical treatments was published in China in 1061. It consisted of around a thousand supposedly effective drugs. Although the original, all twenty-one volumes of it, is lost, many of the entries survive. According to one of these:

> It was said that in order to evaluate the effect of genuine Shangdang ginseng, two persons were asked to run together. One was given the ginseng while the other ran without. After running for approximately three to five li [about a mile] the one without the ginseng developed severe shortness of breath, while the one who took the ginseng breathed evenly and smoothly.

It is the sort of story that sounds convincing. It remains, however, just a story. The trialists and the author mistake the satisfaction of having done an experiment with that of having done a reliable one. It is easy to imagine a host of reasons why one runner might have done better than another in a single trial. But recommendations acquire strength the moment they seem official, or become backed up by reputation or tradition. Beliefs cement themselves in human minds, and getting them out again can be exceedingly difficult.

One belief that people did manage to free themselves of through observation was the use of boiling oil in the treatment of gunshot wounds. Medical opinion in the early sixteenth century was convinced that this was greatly in a patient's interest. Quoted in Donaldson's translation, here is Giovanni da Vigo, surgeon to Pope Julius II, whose surgical textbooks became the standard works from 1514 onwards:

> We have said . . . that the claws and teeth of beasts are venomous and that wounds made by firearms are infected with venom because of the powder and the treatment of the said wounds does not differ greatly. To come quickly to the treatment: if the wound is made by a horse, by a monkey or by a

dog, or by a similar beast and given that the wound is large: one must cauterize the place with oil of elderberry with which should be mixed a little tiriaca galeni [treacle]. And, for wounds made by firearms it suffices to cauterize the place with oil of elderberry or with linseed oil. . .

Ambroise Paré was twenty-seven when he left his Parisian training and went to war. The French armies of François I marched against those of Charles V, the Holy Roman Emperor, and in 1537 Paré joined the French forces as the two armies met near Turin. Here is what he later wrote:

> Now, at that time I was very inexperienced because I had not yet seen the treatment of wounds made by the arquebus; it is true that I had read in the first book of Jean de Vigo about wounds in general, chapter 8, that wounds made by firearms are poisoned because of the powder and for their cure he commands that they be cauterized with oil of elderberry to which a little treacle should be added. Not to fail in the use of this burning oil and knowing that such treatment could be extremely painful for the wounded, I wanted to know before I used it how the other surgeons carried out the first dressing; this they did by applying the said oil as nearly boiling as possible to the wounds so I plucked up courage to do likewise.
>
> At last I ran out of oil and was constrained to apply a digestive made of egg yolk, oil of roses and turpentine. That night I could not sleep easily thinking that by the default in cautery I would find the wounded to whom I had failed to apply the said oil dead of poisoning; and this made me get up at first light to visit them. Beyond my hopes I found those on whom I had put the digestive dressing feeling little pain from their wounds which were not swollen or inflamed, and having

spent quite a restful night. But the others, to whom the said oil had been applied, I found fevered, with great pain and swelling around their wounds.

'*Je le pansay; Dieu le guarit*', he later said. 'I dressed the wound, God healed it.'

Paré, perhaps protected from dogmatism by his own ignorance of Greek and Latin, succeeded in noticing the results of his small natural experiment. It seems unlikely that Paré was the first battlefield surgeon to run out of oil before the end of a bloody day. The salve that he turned to was also one that he had learnt from Vigo's book, but it was one that was meant to be applied some time later, when the wound was already healing. Paré's achievement was to realise that the evidence provided to him by his experience was worth more than the teachings of the greatest known authority. It never occurred to him, though, to deliberately repeat the sort of trial he had blundered into inadvertently, and to test one approach against another intentionally. The thought that the egg yolk, rose oil and turpentine might also be bad for wounds never came to him. (In fact, the dressing was specifically designed to make sure the wound grew infected. The pus of infected wounds was so universal in those unsterile times – appearing without fail as though no wound could mend without it – that doctors believed it was essential for healing.) The closest Paré came to a deliberate trial was when an old woman told him that onion ground up with salt made a good dressing for burns, and he gave it a try:

Some time later a German of the guard of the said seigneur de Montejan [the French infantry commander] was very drunk and his [gunpowder] flask caught fire and caused great damage to his hands and face, and I was called to dress him. I applied onions to one half of his face and the usual remedies to the other. At the second dressing I found the side where I had applied the onions to have no blisters nor scarring and the other side to be all blistered; and so I planned to write about the effects of these onions.

Even today, almost five hundred years after Paré struggled to improve the surgical treatments available to him, it is difficult to keep mentally distinct his unusual successes and his completely ordinary failures. To say he was 'experimenting' with wound dressings implies that he did so in such a way as to be able to tell the difference between what worked and what did not. Since his efforts were not reliable enough to do that, in a sense he was not 'experimenting' at all – he was tinkering, fiddling, messing around, engaged in activities that were fundamentally frivolous in terms of the risks they took with another person's health. As a single attempt, the onions on one part of the face told him nothing. Some wounds heal well, others badly. Infection sometimes strikes here and not there. Only a more methodical and repeated approach could have revealed to Paré if his ground onions held the power to heal.

Our ideas about science have developed, while the words we use to describe them often contain the muddles of half a millennium ago. It would have been better, much better, if the word 'experiment' had come, very strictly, to mean only what was capable of distinguishing between truth and illusion.

John Baptista Van Helmont's book *Oriatrike, or Physick Refined* was published in English in London in 1662, declaring, as textbooks are wont to do, that it set everything right that had been wrong. The book's modest subtitle was: 'The common ERRORS therein REFUTED and the whole ART Reformed & Rectified'. It contained sentiment and imagination of a biblical tendency, both in the style of its prose and the power of its meaning:

For Medicine is not a naked word, a vain boasting, or vain talk, for it leaves a work behind it: Wherefore I despise reproaches, the boastings, and miserable vanities of ambition: Go to, return with me to the purpose: If ye speak truth, Oh ye Schools, that ye can cure any kind of Fevers without evacuation [i.e. using drugs to make people release the contents of their bowels or stomachs], but will not for fear of a worse relapse; come down to the contest ye Humorists [followers of Galen]: Let us take out of the Hospitals, out of the Camps, or from elsewhere, 200, or 500 poor People, that have Fevers, Pleurisies etc. Let us divide them in halves, let us cast lots, that one half of them may fall to my share, and the other to yours; I will cure them without blood-letting and sensible evacuation; but do you do, as ye know . . . we shall see how many Funerals both of us shall have . . .

Unfortunately Van Helmont's strong feelings spent themselves in his words. Had he put in practice the trial that he preached, the world might have changed. Not only might doctors have discovered the harm that they were doing – the evils of taking sick people and bleeding them, giving them diarrhoea or making them vomit – but they might have realised that Van Helmont's technique could help them discover treatments that actually helped. Instead Van Helmont was content with making only a mental experiment, vindicating his ideas to himself only in his own imagination and his bombastic prose. Given that those reading his text could perform the same mental experiment – and, in their own heads, satisfy themselves that *their* patients survived better – Van Helmont persuaded no one. His medicine remained a naked word, and a vain talk, and left no work behind it. The next century, however, was to do better.

5   The Taste of Trees

Opium was not the only drug that eased pain. It was probably not even the commonest. That was alcohol, and it was often more popular with doctors too. The concentration of opium was difficult to predict, and dosing someone by mouth was unreliable. By the time the doctor produced the sedative effect he wanted, the patient might still have a stomach full of the stuff, steadily tipping them beyond peacefulness and into comatose oblivion. Alcohol was less inclined to put people permanently to sleep.

Beyond those two, before the mid-eighteenth century, there was not much else. Cloves had some mild powers, but their cost wasn't matched by their effectiveness. Sugar could help a little. The Jewish practice of giving a baby a teaspoon of sugared wine before a circumcision has been shown to be a significant help – but, unsurprisingly, not a complete one. Edward Stone, born in 1702 to a farming family in Princes Risborough, a town in the Chiltern hills between Oxford and London, was the man who changed things. He went to Oxford at the age of eighteen, before entering the Church. From 1745 he was based in west Oxfordshire, living in the town of Chipping Norton and serving as chaplain to Sir Jonathon Cope at the small village of Breurn. Sometime around 1757, on a walk through the Cotswold countryside, he fell upon an idea.

It began with something that Stone never quite explained. Willow trees grew along the riverbanks, in the fields where he walked. One day he took a piece of bark and put it into his mouth. 'I accidentally tasted it,' he said, rather as though he had tripped over something. Willow bark, Stone discovered, did not have the sweet warmth of cinnamon. In fact, it tasted pretty awful. It was horribly bitter, and it reminded the educated Reverend Stone of something – it reminded him of cinchona.

Looking back, he declared that what motivated him to investigate the bark further was 'the general maxim, that many natural maladies carry their cures along with them, or . . . their remedies lie not far from their causes'. It was a way of thinking packed with unexamined superstition, and not far from the doctrine of signatures that had enthralled Paracelsus and many others. The coincidence of nettles growing alongside the dock leaves that ease their sting was widely noted; the lack of other examples across the breadth of human maladies was overlooked. The Reverend Stone was a firm believer in the Bible and the Church of England. That did not stop him from also holding a few beliefs that were more akin to pagan magic.

Stone reasoned that since malaria was very common in the marshy places where willow grew, it was likely that the tree would cure the disease. That, at least, was how he explained himself six years later. He may have been trying to create a meaningful narrative to impress his audience at the Royal Society. Regardless, it is significant that Stone chose to justify his actions in the way that he did. Technology had developed hugely between early human civilisations and eighteenth-century Oxfordshire: ways of thinking about the world had not necessarily followed.

Seeking to investigate whether willow could be as useful as cinchona, Stone collected the bark one summer, then put it in a bag near a baker's oven. Three months later it was dry enough to be pounded into powder. With malaria common around Chipping Norton, the Reverend began treating people with his new powder. It seemed to work – when he gave it to people, he felt that their fevers went down and that they went on to recover. Whether they would have done so anyway, and possibly sooner if he had left them in peace, did not occur to him. For five more years the Reverend Stone continued to dose the malarial residents of Chipping Norton, before screwing up his courage to write to the Royal Society.

His bark, he said, 'hath been given I believe to fifty persons, and never failed in the cure, except in a few autumnal and quartan agues'. It was exactly the sort of reasoning that Galen had used, describing his remedy that cured absolutely everyone – except for those who died, who must therefore have been incurable.

Cinchona bark had originally been substituted for Peruvian balsam as a way of saving money. It was only good fortune that cinchona turned out, not only to reduce fevers as the balsam had done, but actually to cure malaria. Now Stone had come up with a new money-saving option. Rather than import expensive cinchona from Peru, Englishmen could gather a cheap alternative.

Inasmuch as the dried willow bark actually did reduce fevers, Stone's discovery was a success. He had no way of knowing, given the limitations of the world he lived in, that fever was not itself the disease, but the body's method of trying to fight its way back to health. What he potentially could have grasped, but did not, was that what mattered was not whether patients were feverish and uncomfortable for a few days, but whether, in the end, they survived.

Part of what stopped Stone from thinking about this was that, to his mind, he could see the treatment working. The fevers subsided, the patients generally got better. When someone got worse instead, there was always a reason to hand.

The ancient use of willow had fallen out of favour and none of the books that Stone looked in said much about it. The Egyptians said they used it to give strength to the heart, which it was incapable of doing. They put it on infected ears and aching muscles, into neither of which it was easily absorbed. Dioscorides in AD 100 mentioned the use of willow – but dealt only with the leaves, not the bark that was the rich source of the active ingredient. So the use of willow went back a long way, but in the same style as the medical use of celery and lettuce and watermelon. Stone's achievement was to note a real effect of the bark – its ability to bring down fevers – even though he mistook this for a guarantee of its helping provide a cure.

By the end of the eighteenth century, as Stone had hoped, willow bark was a widespread medication. William White, an apothecary, spoke gratefully about its use. 'Since the introduction of this bark into practice, in the Bath City Infirmary and Dispensary, as a substitute for the Cinchona, not less than 20 pounds a year have been saved to the Charity.' He worked to develop extracts of the bark. When the Napoleonic war made imports more difficult, efforts to replace cinchona increased even further. Willow, which did not cure malaria, thus partly replaced cinchona, which did. Doctors felt pleased at their advance.

6 Beetroots, Mesmerism and Organic Chemistry

Ignorance is a great spur to questioning, and to progress. The physical scientists from the Royal Society onwards were excited to realise how much they did not know, and how much remained to be discovered. Perhaps no group were more enchanted, more enthralled, or more full of promise to the world, than the chemists.

Chemistry had developed from medieval and Renaissance alchemy. The ethos of alchemy was that of the conspiracy theory. Someone, somewhere, had discovered how to turn lead into gold. It was an alchemist's task to uncover the information that others were keeping secret, to root out the heart of the mystery. Clues were to be found everywhere – in coded messages hidden within books, in signs from the heavens. What all alchemists understood was that the knowledge was already out there, squirrelled away. Paranoia went together with a belief in magic: the natural world felt to alchemists like something already fully explored, where the best bits had been hidden by those who had got there first.

Chemistry was born, in the seventeenth and eighteenth centuries, out of a different feeling. Nature was open and honest, its practitioners believed, there for all to explore. Anyone able to devise the right method could be rewarded with understanding. Her mysteries need not be approached secretively. The greater the intelligence you came to her with, the more she would reveal.

It was not until the middle of the eighteenth century that chemistry was able 'to free itself from these delusions, and to venture abroad in all the native dignity of a useful science'. So wrote Thomas Thomson, Regius Professor of Chemistry at Glasgow, in 1830, reviewing the development of his discipline from its alchemical roots. By the middle of the preceding century, he believed, chemists had finally begun 'to be useful to man, by furnishing him with better and more powerful medicines than the ancient physicians were acquainted with'.

Thomson was writing at a time when the realisation of medicine's uselessness had not really dawned. His belief that chemists had extended the range of effective medicines was inaccurate, as was his assumption that there had ever been a substantial range to extend. The ancients had possessed opium, and now there was cinchona and willow bark. None could be credited to chemistry.

Advances, however, had been made, like that of Paracelsus dissolving opium in alcohol rather than water. The next break-through came in the unlikely shape of the beetroot. In the middle of the eighteenth century the German Andreas Sigismund Marggraf found that he could use brandy to extract crystals from this undistin-guished root vegetable. They tasted sweet. Marggraf showed that they were the same substance as that which gave the sweetness to sugar cane. Efforts to breed sweetness into beetroot began. The importance of Marggraf's innovation was his demonstration that what mattered was not where a molecule (in this case sugar) had come from, but the nature of the molecule itself. It was a move towards the idea that a chemical's structure, rather than its heritage, determined its function.

The next step was taken by Antoine François Fourcroy, the son of an apothecary in the service of the Duc d'Orléans. He qualified as a doctor in 1780 and turned his attentions to chemistry, taking up a lecturer's post in the subject four years later. With cinchona bark still in demand, and still exceedingly expensive, efforts were being made to find both replacements and counterfeits. Fourcroy was well connected but from a poor background; his evident talent led the French Société Royale de Médecine to sponsor his medical education. Even before it was finished they were employing him to help analyse mineral waters. Fourcroy responded by developing reagents, substances that reacted with what was in the water, allowing analyses that were not only newly accurate but also did not require the water to be boiled down in order to measure the solids dissolved within it. Impressed by the great French chemist Lavoisier, Fourcroy worked not only to advance his own experiments in chemistry, but also to help others to do the same.

In 1784 Lavoisier was temporarily distracted from his other researches by a request from Louis XVI of France. Franz Mesmer was obtaining impressive medical results by a process that seemed difficult to understand. By sitting close and touching people, he appeared able to heal a range of problems. He felt his healing utilised 'animal magnetism', a heretofore undiscovered physical fluid, one that was simply not apparent to other observers but that connected him with his patients. The king wanted to know if it was real. He set up a commission to investigate, appointing four doctors (including Guillotin, later the inventor of the 'humane' and 'democratic' machine) and five leading scientists, among them Lavoisier and Benjamin Franklin. The commission decided that Mesmer's 'animal magnetism' was a fantasy. This was Lavoisier's opinion:

> The art of concluding from experience and observation consists in evaluating probabilities, in estimating if they are high or numerous enough to constitute proof . . . The success of charlatans, sorcerers, and alchemists – all those who abuse public credulity – is founded on errors of this type of calculation.

Lavoisier was being a bit unfair, since the greatest dangers to public credulity were not from those who set out intentionally to fool people, but from those who had already fooled themselves. Some of those were mesmerists; many more were doctors.

Lavoisier's language is interesting. Reaching conclusions was an 'art', relying on 'experience and observation' rather than experiment. Numerical answers came not by calculation, but by estimate. It was an inadvertently accurate summary of the way even members of the king's commission decided what medical effects were real, and what were not. Irrationality, Lavoisier concluded, was most likely when it came to those things 'that touch the most'. People wanted to know what the future held, and they wanted to prolong their lives. Their desires made them unable to think clearly on those subjects.

In the meantime, Fourcroy's experience in analysing mineral water made him well qualified to approach more solid matters. He undertook an analysis of bark from trees that were being used as alternatives to cinchona. *Cinchona floribunda*, also called Quinquina of St Domingo, was one: its name neatly combining the actions of a hope and an advertisement. Fourcroy published his analysis of the bark's chemical components in 1791. It came to be regarded as a model way of exploring a vegetable substance, but Fourcroy was able to say very little about the bitter-tasting residue that was putatively the bark's active ingredient, and got nowhere in actually isolating an anti-malarial compound.* His success in breaking the bark down into constituent substances, however, prompted interest from others in continuing his approach. Fourcroy encouraged these interests, as did the French government. These early efforts at chemical analysis were driven by concerns over the dilution and adulteration of medical compounds, in particular of opium and cinchona. Commercial interests also pushed development. Once the Napoleonic War was

* The tree was later renamed *Exostemma floribundum*, correctly dismissing any notion that it was a form of cinchona.

blocking trade between France and the tropical British colonies, extracting sugar from beetroot suddenly became financially profitable. It made people think about the value of the chemical processes involved. If you could replace expensive sugar cane imports with something so simple as beetroot, what else could you do? Solvent extraction, the chemist's method for separating and thereby concentrating particular parts of a fluid (or a vegetable), began to seem like a technique with more than academic interest.

From the early years of the nineteenth century, the successful isolation of active drug principles began. At first it was haphazard. In 1803 Charles Derosne, a Parisian pharmacist, while attempting to devise a way of measuring concentrations of opium, ended up with a substance he did not understand and that he found to be peculiarly alkaline. Chemists had learnt to expect that the constituent parts they derived from plants would be acid. Derosne mistakenly put the oddity down to his having contaminated the crystals with potash, and thought no more of it. Around the same time Friedrich Sertürner, a young Austrian apothecary, made a similar discovery. He published on the subject repeatedly from 1805, attracting little attention. Then in 1817 he managed to get his paper into the journal edited by France's leading chemist, Gay-Lussac. *Annales de Chimie* had been founded in 1789 by Lavoisier and continued to attract general interest. Its readers realised these alkaline crystals were something strikingly special.

Gay-Lussac's editorial pointed out that Sertürner had isolated what appeared to be the active ingredient of opium. (Sertürner and three volunteers convincingly demonstrated their case by accidentally overdosing themselves with it.) Sertürner had called it morphium: Gay-Lussac, wishing to make the name reflect the odd fact that the substance was alkaline, altered that to morphine. Yet it was not the achievement of this specific isolation that Gay-Lussac felt was of chief importance. He was more excited by the principle it established, that plants contained something more than the organic acids heretofore isolated. If the first-ever organic alkali was morphine, what else might it be within the power of plants to provide?

Cinchona was an obvious target for this sort of hopeful interest. A few half-successful efforts had been made in the years before Gay-Lussac's editorial, but only after its publication did people begin looking for *alkaline* substances. Once they knew what they were after, progress was quick. In 1820 the Frenchmen Pelletier and Caventou isolated quinine. It turned out to be one of a number of substances in cinchona bark that had anti-fever and anti-malarial properties. Pelletier and Caventou understood that these newly uncovered plant ingredients might be of wider use. They recommended that they be properly investigated for their direct medical uses.

To an extent, the discovery of what came to be called alkaloids helped medicine take its ignorance more seriously. Chemistry was developing new drugs, different from anything that had gone before. You did not have to suggest that your teachers and your idols might have been mistaken in order to believe that the effects of these novel medicines might not be fully worked out.

The development of pharmacopoeias whose ingredients were chemicals rather than plants was a boon. The properties of plants varied so much, between seasons and climates and even plots of earth, that notions of testing were handicapped by the difficulty of obtaining consistent drugs. Quinine was a lot more palatable and a lot less noxious than the cinchona bark which contained a lot of other alkaloids as well. People swallowed quinine with more success than cinchona, and vomited it up again less frequently. Our modern fantasy of the gentle benevolence of plants, and the acrid artificiality of drugs, was inconceivable to these early pioneers, who saw things very much the other way around. The birth of the modern pharmaceutical industry began with efforts to convert ever-increasing amounts of the natural bark to the gentler and more effective sulphate of quinine.

In the ten years from 1828, progress was made in isolating active compounds that could replace willow bark. In Germany, Italy and in France salicin (from the Latin name for willow, *Salix*) and then salicylic acid were developed. They, too, quickly became used as substitutes for the continually expensive cinchona and its modern derivative of quinine. Like willow bark, neither salicin nor salicylic acid had any anti-malarial activity.

It was in 1828, also, that Friedrich Wöhler synthesised urea. The molecule by which humans get rid of nitrogen, urea is an essential part of the way our bodies handle proteins, and a key waste molecule in urine. It also contains carbon and is therefore organic. Yet Wöhler made it out of ammonium cyanate, an entirely inorganic compound. For the first time chemists knew that they were able to artificially construct a molecule that previously had existed only as the product of a living creature.

7 New England and New Ways of Thinking

Mental techniques as well as chemical ones were advancing.

Born in Cambridge, Massachusetts, at the start of the nineteenth century, Oliver Wendell Holmes contemplated abandoning medicine for poetry. At the age of twenty-one, his poem 'Old Ironsides' won him national attention. It was written to celebrate the wooden-hulled American warship, a veteran of the 1812 war against the British, built from American live oaks and clad in copper by the Revolutionary hero Paul Revere. The success of the poem touched Holmes's imagination; he spoke of the 'lead poisoning' that entered his soul on seeing his own words in print.

Against his inclination to art, however, was the Calvinist devotion to work in which he had been raised. Poetry was an admirable talent for a cultured man, but a suspect occupation for his entire career. After a thoroughly American elite education – Phillips Academy followed by Harvard – Holmes went to Paris in 1833, at the age of twenty-four. For a while he spent his time at the races and the theatre. Then, his puritan side winning through, he concentrated on his studies at the École de Médecine. There he came under the influence of the nation's leading teacher, Pierre Charles Alexandre Louis.

Louis harboured an unusual scepticism about the value of existing medical knowledge. The accepted theory was that a fever resulted from inflammation, from an excess of blood: attaching leeches

71

closest to the inflamed bit of the body drew this away, easing the fever; in pneumonia, for example, the leeches were put on the patient's chest. In addition to their own indigenous supply, in the year that Holmes arrived in Paris the French medical industry imported an *extra* forty-two million leeches. Hungary and the Ukraine, Turkey, Romania, Russia and North Africa were exporters. And with a lifespan of almost a decade, the leeches were highly reusable.

Seemingly it was inconceivable for anyone to consider that all bleeding was useless or, worse, harmful. Yet Louis questioned the way in which people were bled, and came up with new ideas as well as, more significantly, setting out thoughtfully to test them. 'What was to be done,' he asked, 'in order to know whether blood-letting had any favourable influence on pneumonia, and the extent of that influence?' It was a question much on his mind during the time that Holmes studied under him. Louis's first attempt to write on the subject was an 1828 article, which led to a full-blown book in 1835. What Louis wanted to clarify was *when* patients should be bled. Was it best to attach the leeches to their chests on the day they fell ill? The day after? The day after that? What troubled him was the knowledge that each patient was different, and that their fitness and their age and the severity of their infection could all vary. How, he wondered, could he avoid mistaking the influence of these factors for the influence of his leeches?

The gradual development of our ability to think clearly about such issues is not a sequence of precisely linked events. Louis did not think as he did because he read Van Helmont, nor were Holmes's later thoughts the direct products of his time in France. These inventive thinkers, arriving at ways of seeing the world that were more correct and useful than what had come before, advanced the progress of human culture with ideas that were partly their own and partly not. Ideas about truth, about experimental method and how science could best discover Nature were bubbling under, bursting forth now in one person's way of looking at the world and now another's.

For any particular disease, wrote Louis,

> let us suppose five hundred of the sick, taken indiscriminately, are subjected to one kind of treatment, and five hundred others, taken in the same manner, are treated in a different mode; if the mortality is greater among the first than among the second, must we not conclude that the treatment was less appropriate, or less efficacious, in the first class than in the second?

What had been only carelessly implied in Van Helmont's description in 1662 was thoughtfully exposed in Louis's. The natural differences between one patient and another, between this instance of infection and that, could be prevented from biasing a test's results by simply including a large enough group of people and spreading them randomly. As Louis acknowledged:

> It is impossible to appreciate each case with mathematical exactness, and it is precisely on this account that enumeration becomes necessary. By so doing, the errors (which are inevitable) being the same in the two groups of patients subjected to different treatments, mutually compensate each other, and they may be disregarded without materially affecting the exactness of the results.

In other words, it doesn't matter that everyone is different so long as you take a large enough group of people and spread them out randomly. Some will be sicker than others, some healthier. Take enough of them and the differences will balance out. Louis had discovered the cure for the mental error that the Chinese had made almost a millennium before, racing one man dosed with ginseng against another who was not and concluding that the drug accounted for all the differences between them.

Louis went on to make a stronger point. Given that people are different, and the diseases that grip them also vary, what alternative is there to averaging out those differences with large numbers? The alternative is to pretend that your own judgement is capable of noticing and correctly accounting for all the differences that exist, and pretending none of them can bias your intuitions or undermine your conclusions. Avoiding numbers did not mean that you avoided being misled by the natural differences between patients, only that you avoided acknowledging them. Race two people against each other, or even ten, and one group might be naturally faster than the other. Race a random 500 against a random 500 more and you could reasonably expect the groups to have a similar performance.

Like Van Helmont's, however, Louis's ideas were better than his practice. He never did take 500 of the sick, and allocate one portion of them to one treatment and the rest to another. Instead he took the records of seventy-seven patients previously diagnosed with pneumonia, then looked at what happened to them relative to the length of the delay before bleeding was begun. Louis's study, for all his good qualities, was woefully limited. The patients were not spread by chance, nor allocated to different approaches. They were selected after the event, and compared to others that Louis thought looked pretty similar. His conclusions, as a result, were not useful, and his failure to make the most of the methods he suggested limited his influence for good.

It was no coincidence, though, that Louis's belief in testing went along with a scepticism about the value of medical interventions. Oliver Wendell Holmes returned to Boston soaked in both of these new beliefs. At Harvard he became both Professor of Anatomy and Professor of Physiology (less of a chair, he commented, and more of an entire settee). He also took up a more informal position as one of the nation's leading intellectuals, a Boston Brahmin and friend of men like Henry Wadsworth Longfellow, William Cullen Bryant, John Greenleaf Whittier and James Russell Lowell. In their company he continued writing, regularly publishing poems and prose in the *Atlantic Monthly* and in books like *The Autocrat at the Breakfast Table*.

From February 1843 Holmes helped pioneer the idea that puerperal fever, then a leading cause of maternal death, was actually spread to women by their medical attendants. Puerperal fever was a wound infection, the result of bacteria taking hold in the raw lining of the womb after a woman's child was born. Holmes was not the first to notice that it was chiefly spread by doctors, but he was one of the first to publicly argue his case. It was a conclusion that doctors could have reached far sooner, if only they were not so wedded to their belief in their own benevolence. 'Doctors are gentlemen', said Charles Meigs, a leading obstetrician who was too appalled by Holmes's suggestion to take it seriously, 'and gentlemen's hands are clean.' Meigs was neither stupid nor ill-meaning, just reliant on his belief that well-educated and compassionate doctors must, by their virtues, bring their patients health and healing.

Holmes thought differently. 'In my own family,' he wrote, 'I had rather that those I esteemed the most should be delivered unaided, in a stable, by the mangerside, than that they should receive the best help, in the fairest apartment, but exposed to the vapors of this pitiless disease.' Having been schooled in uncertainty, he found the idea that doctors could sometimes cause harm perfectly reasonable.

In May 1860, Holmes addressed the Massachusetts Medical Society. He gave them a blunt verdict on the value of their mutual practices. 'I firmly believe that if the whole materia medica, *as now used*, could be sunk to the bottom of the sea, it would be all the better for mankind, and all the worse for the fishes.'

'Materia medica' meant all the drugs that mankind possessed. In Holmes's view doctors were better off leaving well alone. Their job was to support the patients emotionally, to encourage them in sensible and healthy habits, and to admit that all the 'cures' and 'treatments' that civilisation had so far devised amounted, when put together, to poisons.

He spoke about what he thought were the causes of the situation. His descriptions of mental errors were similar to Bacon's, and he quoted Bacon while talking of them. As well as the errors of thought in reasoning about human health, though, Holmes also spoke of the culture of medicine-taking. 'Somebody buys all the quack medicines that build palaces for the . . . millionaires [who make them]. Who is it? These people have a constituency of millions. The popular belief is all but universal that sick persons should feed on noxious substances.' A society, he was saying, gets the doctors it deserves. If people cry out for medical attendants who will drug them at every opportunity, that is what they get. And Americans were even more gullible than citizens of quieter and less successful nations. Americans, said Holmes, loved extravagance

> . . . in remedies and trust in remedies, as in everything else. How could a people which has a revolution once in four years [i.e. an elected change of government], which has contrived the Bowie-knife and the revolver, which has chewed the juice out of all the superlatives in the language in Fourth of July orations . . . which insists on sending out yachts and horses and boys to out-sail, out-run, out-fight, and checkmate all the rest of creation; how could such a people be content with any but 'heroic' practice? What wonder that the stars and stripes wave over doses of ninety grains of quinine, and that the American eagle screams with delight to see three drachms of calomel given at a single mouthful?

Doctors, wishing to be successful as much as they wished to be helpful, played up to it all, 'loving to claim as much for our art as we can'. Holmes's feeling that medicine did more harm than good was not unique. Here is Samuel Hahnemann, a German physician fifty years older than Holmes, describing his feelings on realising that the treatments available to him at the end of the eighteenth century were harmful:

> My sense of duty would not easily allow me to treat the unknown pathological state of my suffering brethren with these unknown medicines. The thought of becoming in this way a murderer or malefactor towards the life of my fellow human beings was most terrible to me, so terrible and disturbing that I wholly gave up my practice in the first years of my married life and occupied myself solely with chemistry and writing.

Hahnemann's desperation to get out of this situation, 'so terrible and disturbing', led him to seek for certainties. Overdosing himself with cinchona, in an experiment that began with no hypothesis, Hahnemann made himself so ill that his symptoms resembled those of malaria. His conclusion was that a drug 'which can produce a set of symptoms in a healthy individual, can treat a sick individual who is manifesting a similar set of symptoms'. Combined with a fantasy that water could contain the 'memory' of a substance that had once been in it, Hahnemann invented homeopathy.*

Oliver Wendell Holmes devoted a considerable portion of his mental and literary energy to attacking homeopathy, a way of thinking that angered him. Replacing mistakes with delusions, said

---

* I am using the word 'fantasy' deliberately, to signify that what Hahnemann developed was not a theory. It was not a theory becuase it was not something that he attempted to test or could conceive of disproving.

Holmes, was not a valiant way of facing up to the uncertainties, mysteries and doubts with which mankind was surrounded.

Towards the end of his life, Oliver Wendell Holmes was asked a curious question. It came from William Osler, the Canadian physician who rose, largely on the charisma of his personality, to become the most popular doctor of the nineteenth century. Osler wanted to know what had given Holmes more satisfaction – his medicine or his poetry. In other words, had he made the right decision, abandoning his ambitions to become a poet in order to practise physic?

With puritan grace, Holmes answered that undoubtedly his medicine mattered most. He had tried to save lives, if only by educating doctors about the harms they were inflicting on their patients. But he quickly turned to his memories of writing poetry. 'I was filled with a better feeling, the highest state of mental exaltation and the most crystalline clairvoyance that had ever been granted to me – I mean that lucid vision of one's thought and all forms of expression which will be at once precise and musical.'

Being useful to your fellow men was what an elite member of the nineteenth-century Boston intelligentsia knew should matter most. All the same, it was never quite where Holmes's heart lay.

Osler's own greatest achievement was to spur doctors into a belated sense of their own inadequacies. His textbook, *The Principles and Practice of Medicine*, a bestseller around the start of the twentieth century, pointed out that understanding of diseases had developed tremendously, but the medical ability to intervene had not. By then the world was readier to hear such messages, and Osler's view of the world was greeted as exciting and full of promise. The Rockefeller Foundation, later to sponsor huge amounts of clinically useful medical research, was set up partly in response to the opportunities highlighted by Osler's book.

The advances of Holmes and of Louis, the mental methods that they successfully popularised, led to no immediate new therapies. But they paved the way for doctors to begin understanding the limitations of those they possessed, and the need to improve. And the next innovation, when it came, arrived from an unexpected direction: dyestuffs.

8 Dyes, Stains and Antibiotics

The origins of modern drugs are profoundly mixed up with our interest in brightly coloured cloths and fabrics, and with the dyes that produced them. These dyes, in turn, derived from an accidental by-product of a new invention: gaslight.

In the 1790s, the inventor William Murdoch, working to help industrialise the Cornish tin mines, found that if coal was heated within an enclosed space, it gave off a flammable gas, one that 'burnt with great brilliancy'. By 1794 his house in Redruth was being lit by this 'gaslight'. By 1807 so was Pall Mall in London. Westminster Bridge followed in 1813, then the city of Baltimore in 1816, then Paris in 1820. Over the next few years Murdoch's gaslight began shining out from the world's most developed towns.

England, rich in coal, was not alone in finding that this wonderful new process had an unwanted consequence: a sticky, smelly waste residue called coal tar.

The German chemist Friedrich Runge, in 1834, was working with benzene. Benzene was one of the constituents of coal tar, by that stage a rapidly multiplying and unwanted commodity. Runge treated benzene with chloride of lime and produced a colour so blue that he named the substance cyanol. Other chemists made similar discoveries, giving them different names. In 1855 the German chemist August Wilhelm von Hofmann, looking at all these compounds, realised that they were the same thing. He called them aniline.

Possibly the implications of their colour should have occurred to him, as it also should have to Friedrich Runge. Hofmann admired the colour of his coal-tar-derived aniline, then moved on to studying more important aspects of it than its prettiness.

Brought to England in 1845 at the behest of Prince Albert, Hofmann was the founding director of London's new Royal College of Chemistry. His chemical 'first love' was aniline. The nature of it fascinated him, partly because of the way in which related chemicals had shared properties. This raised the tantalising possibility that their molecular structures – if such things could be worked out – would show similarities that corresponded to and explained their external and chemical ones. Benzene, derived from coal tar by one of Hofmann's English students, was at the core of the family of molecules that included aniline, and which Hofmann called 'aromatic'. He gave them the name because they smelt sweet.

Techniques for determining the structure of molecules were primitive, but chemists were effective at figuring out the elements that composed them. Benzene, for example, was C_6H_6, although the way those carbons and hydrogens fitted together was a mystery.* Hofmann, like many before him, wanted to synthesise quinine. In an 1849 report to the Royal College of Chemistry, he suggested that:

> . . . it is obvious that napthalidine, differing only by the elements of two equivalents of water, might pass into [quinine] simply by an assumption of water. We cannot, of course, expect to induce the water to enter merely by placing it in context, but a happy experiment may attain this end . . .

Four years after this, a fifteen-year-old boy named William Perkin came to study under Hofmann at the Royal College. For a youngster

---

* One famously solved by Kekulé dreaming of a snake swallowing its own tail, then waking to the realisation that benzene was a ring.

fascinated by the possibilities of chemistry, there was no mentor better. Not only was Hofmann brilliant, full of love for colleagues and chemicals alike, but his love and his brilliancy were catching. 'Who would not work, and even slave, for Hofmann?' recalled another student. 'There was an indescribable charm in working with Hofmann, in watching his delight at a new result or his pathetic momentary depression when failure attended the attempt to attain a result which theory indicated. "Another dream is gone," he would mutter plaintively, with a deep sigh.'

The natural world that Hofmann lived in was full of wonders. Perkin remembered him wandering around the laboratory happily, admiring the new compounds that were everywhere being derived for the first time, and joining in his students' explorations. 'Taking a little of the substance in a watch glass, he treated it with caustic alkali, and at once obtained a beautiful scarlet salt. Looking up at us in his characteristic and enthusiastic way, he at once exclaimed, Gentlemen, new bodies are floating in the air!'

It is difficult, living in a world that holds 'artificial' as a pejorative, to imagine how fresh and wonderful these colours seemed, the extent to which 'artificiality' meant a fertile combination of human talents and Nature's richness. Chemistry had the potential to offer compounds of power, and the attractions for the chemists were aesthetic as well as intellectual. Perkin and a friend, Arthur Church, were both keen painters. Colours attracted them and aroused their curiosity. While Hofmann viewed colour as something interesting for its chemical implications, Perkin and Church saw it as important in itself. In 1856 they submitted to the Royal Society a report 'On Some New Colouring Matters'. Distillations gave them oranges and crimsons and dark yellows, 'with a lustre somewhat similar to that of murexide'.

Murexide was a curious substance. The original source was a cone-shaped marine snail of the genus *Murex*, which could be crushed to release tiny quantities of a precious purple dye. (An old myth told of Hercules walking his dog on the shore of the Mediterranean and the dog chewing snails and staining its mouth.) The Romans treasured it, not least because of its rarity – over 10,000 snails were needed to colour a single toga. The German chemist Carl Wilhelm Scheele described making murexide artificially in 1776 from the uric acid of human kidney and bladder stones. Then the doctor William Prout, much interested in the medical problems such stones caused, found that an even richer source for uric acid was the excrement of boa constrictors. (Reptiles, like birds, excrete their protein waste in a more concentrated form than mammals.) By chemical transformation Prout arrived at ammonium purpurate, and he called it murexide for the purple colour that so resembled that of the Phoenician sea snails. By analogy, he suggested that murexide might be useful as a dye – but that was as far as the idea went.

'I was ambitious enough to want to work on this subject,' said Perkin, about Hofmann's dream of making quinine from the coal tar residue napthalidine. He spent his spare hours during the spring and summer of 1856 in a room on the top floor of his father's East End house. Wreathed in the stink of ammonia, surrounded by his experiments in painting and photography, on a desk stained by all his various efforts, he changed the world.

Attempting to produce quinine, which was known to be colour-less, Perkins ended up with something red. Wanting to understand where he had gone wrong, he tried a similar experiment using aniline as his starting material. This time he got something that was impressively black, then, after rinsing out the flask he had made it in, he noticed that the alcohol wash left a colour of startling hue and radiance. Perkin had produced mauve.

He found that his colour stained silk, and that the newly mauve fabric kept its appearance despite being washed and hung up in the sun. At the end of August he filed a patent, and started to explore the potential for his discovery as a commercial dye. It exploded.

Queen Victoria wore mauve to her eldest daughter's wedding in 1858, then again in 1862 when she swept into the Great London Exhibition. In between, Charles Dickens's *All the Year Round* said Perkin's mauve made Tyrian purple look 'tame, dull and earthy'. It was part of a craze for the colour that made Perkin's fortune, stimulating the development of a synthetic dye industry that aimed to take advantage of the rainbow of colours hidden within coal tar. Perkin himself went on to develop Britannia Violet, Perkin's Green, and a method for commercially producing a brilliant red. Others rushed in with yellows and violets, blues and browns and blacks and every shade around them. By 1863 there was even a range of different magentas, named for their inventor: the Hofmann Violets, a belated contribution by the man who had initially failed to see the commercial importance of colourings. This was the new and wholly unexpected world of chemistry; imperial and potent and pregnant with synthetic power.

The impact of the artificial dyes was vast, not only in terms of fashion and economics but also in stimulating the development of organic chemistry. What had been an academic field became of immense industrial importance. This was scientific progress that people could *see*, a visible and vivid reminder of the power of invention, and the promise it held to add colour to people's lives.

Worries about toxicity developed early, partly in response to the real danger posed by arsenic in the manufacture of some dyes. These concerns were almost immediately exaggerated into a widespread belief that all aniline dyes, and possibly all the products of chemists and factories everywhere, were inherently poisonous. Brewers in the north of England discovered that beer made from Thames water had a pleasantly bitter taste by virtue of a molecule it picked up from the river. Picric acid, the molecule in question, began to be added by northern brewers to produce the same effects. Even as chemists were able to establish molecular similarities – to show that picric acid added to Burton beer was the same as that which the waters of the Thames added in London – people were wondering if a molecule's power lay not in its structure but in its provenance, whether beer with naturally acquired picric acid was safer than when someone had tipped the ingredient in from a flask.

Most of the key steps in the developing dye industry were British. Faraday found benzene, Mansfield showed how to make it on a large scale from coal tar, Perkin and other of his compatriots came up with many of the early colours. Despite it all, in the wake of Prince Albert's death in 1861 Hofmann found that the British were not really interested in science at all, except as an amateur hobby. He returned to Germany. The British chemists that he left behind were struck by their country's lack of interest in encouraging competitive commercialisation of new chemical products. Britain began losing its early lead to German competition.

During the second half of the nineteenth century, Germany led in both industrial chemistry and medical research. Bismarck Brown rapidly joined Britannia Violet in the new pantheon of colours. The industry that Perkin founded in London was adopted far more vigorously on the banks of the Rhine than the Thames. Conducive patent laws, government encouragement and more thoughtful entrepreneurs all helped. Vital, also, was the contempt that scientifically minded Britons tended to feel for commercialising their work. 'England is not the land of science,' said a German delegate to the 1837 Liverpool conference of the British Association for the Advancement of Science. It worshipped the gentleman amateur to a damaging degree. 'There is only widespread dilettantism, [English] chemists are ashamed to be known by that name because it has been assumed by the apothecaries, who are despised.'

By 1879 there were seventeen dye-works in Germany, and only six in England. When the First World War broke out, Germany was supplying three quarters of the world's dyes. England, despite having given birth to the industry, was importing from Germany 80 per cent of what it needed.

The immediate importance of dyes to medical research was through their power to expose the processes of both health and disease. The history of their use in this way was already old. In 1566, madder, the ancient vegetable dye, was noted to stain the bodies of the sheep that fed on it. An animal's bones turned red. Just over a hundred years later Raymond Vieussens, a French anatomist, was injecting saffron brandy into the necks of animals, pushing it into their carotid arteries to see which bits of their brains changed colour.

At the same time, in England, Robert Hooke was using his 'sharpen'd Pen-knife' to cut thin slices of cork. He went on to examine them with the use of a new tool, the microscope. Leeuwenhoek's demonstration of 'animalcules' with the microscope should have alerted the world to something important. Here was the opportunity to understand crucial new things about the way in which life worked. Had it sparked the interest it deserved, it could have led to the acceptance of germ theory centuries ahead of Pasteur. A few years after Robert Hooke sliced cork, Leeuwenhoek was doing the same. Contact with the Royal Society of which Hooke was a part gave Leeuwenhoek an audience for his research. A letter from Leeuwenhoek to the Royal Society in 1674 had some of his preparations attached to it – thin pieces of cork, of quill, of elder and 'the optic nerve of a cow'.

In a later letter, from 1714, Leeuwenhoek told the Royal Society about his efforts to combine such slices with coloured stains. Like Vieussens, Leeuwenhoek used saffron. He wanted to compare the muscle of a fat cow with that of a thin one, and wrote that:

Since the fibres, cut into the thinnest possible layers, were so transparent that they could hardly be recognised, I have macerated a little crocus in brandy. To make the flesh particles more visible to the artist, I have merely moistened them with this wine, whereupon they were bright with a yellow colour.

Not many people read Leeuwenhoek's letter, then or after. A Harvard anatomist, Frederick Lewis, coming upon it during the Second World War, was so excited by the discovery that he repeated the experiment, simmering some saffron up in Boston tap water before applying it to a thinly sliced piece of steak and finding that 'the fibers indeed glow with a golden yellow color'.

People had been adding dyes to the soil and water of plants for a long time before – turning lilies red with powdered cinnabar, or using saffron to make roses yellow – but it was not until the early 1700s that Nicolas Sarrabat, a Jesuit priest and natural philosopher in Lyons, made use of the technique to try to determine how plants worked. He used the Mexican pokeweed berry, finding that its colour penetrated the smallest branches of the roots. When the plant under investigation was washed, the stain remained, visibly outlining the portions of the roots where the absence of its epidermis, the plant's skin, allowed the transfer of nutrients and water.

Despite these hints, people were slow to catch on that a dye's ability to stain selective parts of an organism provided a window onto life's inner workings. Intrigued by madder, in 1736 the British surgeon John Belchier sat down to eat a pig that had been fed on the stuff. The bones and the teeth were red. 'Neither the fleshy nor cartilaginous parts', he recorded, 'suffered the least alteration in colour or in taste.'

Attempts over the following twenty years to selectively dye plant structures led to mixed success. Charles Bonnet, a Swiss lawyer with an active interest in science, used madder and rose and black ink to stain the roots of peas and beans. His efforts, he judged, were 'only weak attempts', but the method was 'a rich mine'. He put camphor in brandy and infused it into a living pear – the leaves took on the camphor's scent, but the fruit seemed not to. After reading Bonnet's 1754 work *Recherches sur l'usage des feuilles dans les plantes*, a medical student named Georg Christian Reichel showed that he could use red stains to prove that the spiral ducts of a plant distributed sap rather than air.

From here on interest accelerated. An English doctor, John Hill, used both cochineal and lead to substantiate his 1770 work *The Construction of Timber*. The vessels by which trees distributed the fluids essential for their lives could, by means of staining, be 'beautifully seen'. Hill developed a machine for cutting sections of his stained wood, a great improvement on Hooke's sharpened penknife, as well as ways of stiffening and blanching the slices that needed it.

Wilhelm Friedrich von Gleichen, who converted his unpromising beginnings to a career of courtly and military success, spent the second part of his life on science. Moved by the work of John Hill and by Leeuwenhoek's animalcules, in 1777 he showed that indigo and cochineal could illuminate the world of these microscopic creatures:

> The bones of animals coloured by the feeding of madder roots led me to this idea. So I coloured some water with carmine, and mixed it with an infusion of wheat in which a swarm of the largest ear-drop organisms and small oval animalcules had been living some months.

The animalcules might be small, but von Gleichen felt that their take-up of the dye was proof that, in some manner at least, they ate and drank like larger creatures. It was a discovery advanced in 1830 when

Christian Gottfried Ehrenberg figured out that only certain dyes were suitable for living creatures: 'These experiments', he noted, 'require organic dyestuffs.' The lead and other substances that dyers often used were too frequently fatal to the animals he wished to study.

Plant experiments dominated, but as the nineteenth century wore on, interest in using stains on larger animals grew. In 1851 the Marquis Alfonso Corti used a carmine dye to illuminate the structure of the inner ear. 'Under the microscope, I found that all its tissue was coloured red, being darker where it was thicker. The holes were clearly seen as small oval windows. I could easily be sure that there was really no tissue in the holes, and I could make out their borders with perfect distinctness.' He was describing the minute holes down which nerves travelled, holes being revealed for the first time by the stain. Carmine, pointed out the marquis, showed up the nuclei of cells. It was an observation of great potential, and situated as it was 'in a great paper in an important German journal' it should have won attention. Instead, in a mid-nineteenth-century world where anatomy, physiology and chemistry were increasingly dominated by the successful Germans, 'it attracted no notice: [since] it was written in French'.

Looking at the names of those who were working in microscopy, you get an impression of the reasons for much of the German success. The work there was being done by professionals, greatly supported by academies and universities. England relied on hobbyists. Lord Osborne demonstrated the staining of wheat cell nuclei to London's Microscopical Society in 1857, while pointing out that as a 'mere amateur' he 'made no attempt to resolve any question in chemistry'. The same year, Hermann Welcker, the gifted German doctor and anatomist, showed the value of stains in illuminating the nuclei of cells in frogs. Leading authors in England and elsewhere heard about Welcker's findings even as Osborne's failed to reach them.

*

Adolf von Baeyer was fascinated by dyes from a young age. He dallied with physics and mathematics as a student at the University of Berlin, then went back to chemistry. From 1856 he was working for Bunsen in Heidelberg, and from the next year for Kekulé, of the benzene-ring dream, in Heidelberg and then in Ghent. From 1866, responding to the urging of Hofmann, the University of Berlin appointed von Baeyer as a senior lecturer, giving him no money but plentiful lab space. He worked on dyes, developing several new classes of chemical and industrial importance. Success, including a Nobel Prize in 1905, firmed rather than dissolved his belief in the essential humility required of a man in possession of theories rather than evidence. Those who designed experiments simply to confirm their prejudices were in danger, he felt, of designing bad ones, of misinterpreting their results, or even of fatally convincing themselves that their theories were too good to need such testing. 'I have never set up an experiment to see whether I was right,' said von Baeyer, 'but to see how the materials behave.'

Methylene blue is an aniline dye. In its powdered form it is a dark deep green; diluted in fluid it looks something like a clear and hopeful sky. It was discovered in 1876 by Heinrich Caro (involved in the development of Bismarck Brown) in collaboration with Baeyer. Caro was laboratory director at Badische Anilin & Soda-Fabrik – BASF. Set up in 1865 in response to the great opportunities for industrial chemistry in Germany, BASF's patent on methylene blue was Germany's first on a coal tar dye, and it became crucially important, through the work of Robert Koch and Paul Ehrlich, in the development of modern medicine.

Pasteur performed marvels in France in the 1860s, persuading the world of the truth of germ theory. A host of incomprehensible diseases were suddenly made clear by the idea of infection, the notion that invisible micro-organisms could invade the body and turn health into illness. Here was suddenly a key to understanding, preventing and potentially treating a host of diseases in previously unthought-of ways.

Despite Pasteur's start, it was once more in Germany that the new techniques really shone. Robert Koch found the organism that caused anthrax in 1877, tuberculosis in 1882 and cholera in 1883. He even developed rules for other microbe hunters: 'Koch's postulates' – intellectual devices for reliably tying together diseases with their causative micro-organisms. Together with a climate of support for seriously conducted science, Germany forged ahead.

One of those supported and inspired by Koch was Paul Ehrlich. He was born in 1854, in Strehlen, Upper Silesia – then part of Prussia, now Poland – and his childhood passions were tied up with this new discipline of microbiology. As a schoolboy he tinkered with microscopes and was introduced to tissue-staining by his cousin, Karl Weigert, whose Breslau laboratory he later worked in. Weigert showed him how aniline dyes could colour cells and tissues, revealing their structure and relationships. Ehrlich was enthralled, 'awakened', as he later remembered, 'to the love and understanding of dyes that have accompanied me throughout my career'. He pursued the subject for his doctorate. Classmates remembered him as the man with the multi-coloured fingers. Over the next five years he used his dyes to explore blood cells, then bacteria. Frustrated after a time with injecting dyes into dead creatures, Ehrlich further developed 'vital staining', showing how methylene blue and other dyes could be injected into, as well as ingested by, living creatures. With encouragement, Ehrlich found, Nature not only showed her secrets, but did so in the most glorious of colours:

If a small quantity of methylene blue is injected into a frog, and a small piece of the tongue is excised and examined, one sees the finest twigs of the nerves beautifully stained, a magnificent dark blue, against a colourless background.

It was Koch who showed how to use methylene blue to stain the tubercle bacillus. With the right dyes the cause of tuberculosis, this ancient and terrible disease, was not only discovered; it was displayed to the world in hues of beautiful pink and blue. Ehrlich was present at the meeting when Koch announced his discovery, and sat close enough to notice what years of work had done to Koch's hands. Their skin was dark and wrinkled, damaged by the stains and disinfectants that the tasks required. Ehrlich listened to Koch's announcement in wonder. 'I hold that evening', he said later, 'to be the most important experience of my scientific life.'

That was in 1882. Largely unwelcome in Berlin's Charité Hospital, where neither his ideas nor his Judaism were popular, Ehrlich became ill. Nevertheless he refined Koch's technique, and, in 1887, used the latest techniques to prove to himself that the spittle he was coughing up contained the tubercle bacillus. The discovery of the bug had not yet led to treatments. Ehrlich went to Egypt, hoping the climate would help his lungs heal. Two years later he returned, feeling somewhat better, this time to work as an assistant at Koch's new Institute for Infectious Diseases.

In Koch's laboratory, Ehrlich was at the heart of the world of medical research – a world that was still small. August von Wasserman, who found his own success researching syphilis, remembered the excitement of the concentration of talents:

If a comparison of any sort is appropriate among such great men, I have to say that Paul Ehrlich was the champagne among the wines. While Koch appeared as the eternally serious-minded academic who thoughtfully weighed and stressed every word, disdaining all theory, observing only what was factual, and describing it in studied terseness, Ehrlich was literally bubbling over with brilliant ideas and views . . .

Ehrlich's laboratory, lined with the palette of his aniline dyes, was a startling sight. 'The visitor was confronted with a symphony of colours,' said Wasserman:

> without exaggeration, thousands upon thousands of glass bottles stood around, all filled with the brightest aniline dyes. Ehrlich . . . was involved in a highly stimulating exchange of ideas with the coal-tar industry. Thus, the industry sent him a sample of each new dye as soon as it appeared, and it was from that time onwards that his lifelong friendships and profound admiration for the creative geniuses and great names in the German dye industry derived.

For a time, Ehrlich left his beloved dyes behind, concentrating instead on the way in which animals seemed able to fight off infection. Serum is the name given to the fluid that blood moves in, the clear liquid turned red by the cells it contains. By exposing animals to infections, then bleeding them, Ehrlich found that their serum developed healing properties. Something in it contained the ingredients of immunity.

Serum therapy set Ehrlich wondering again about his coloured stains. It was clear that something in serum worked as an anti-toxin, specifically capable of fighting off infections like tetanus and diphtheria. These 'antibodies' must work, Ehrlich reasoned, something in the manner of 'magic bullets', ones with the power to find a particular target and destroy only that. He described, sketchily but for the first time, the way living cells could produce antibodies. A letter from 1901, arguing that Ehrlich should be awarded the inaugural Nobel Prize for medicine, noted that his 'explanation is vastly different and much more innovative than anything that has been thought or written on the origin of antibodies so far'. It was, despite that, only one amongst a large number of deeply original pieces of work, including Ehrlich's 'earlier haematological work, the *discovery of the mast cells*, the histo-chemical staining of living nerve fibres with methylene blue, [and] his *vital staining*'. In the event the award of medicine's first Nobel was blocked by a chemist who incorrectly disagreed with some of Ehrlich's ideas, and who disliked the 'markedly Jewish atmosphere' he created.

When Ehrlich injected living rats with methylene blue, he found that the dye was taken up particularly by nerve cells. The stain had some selectivity for that bit of the body, a property that reminded Ehrlich of the manner in which antibodies seemed to pick out their targets. He set out to find chemicals that would work in the same way, mimicking the body's own ability to fight off infection, binding themselves only to the infecting organisms and killing only them.

It is easy to get an impression of Ehrlich as a man consumed with microbes and chemicals, just as it is straightforward to imagine that these successful new doctors were less concerned with individual suffering than their less effective predecessors of generations before. Neither impression is true. Ehrlich was neither cold nor consumed with any imaginary omnipotence. He knew that his tuberculosis might come back at any point, and that there was little anyone could do about it. And he worked in the wards as well as the laboratories.

Whoever has seen Paul Ehrlich at a sickbed in one of the spreading wards of a large hospital, must have noticed that this extraordinary man embodied the humanist as physician. I was touched by the tenderness with which he took care of his child patients, how he joked with them and tried to soothe their discomfort by caresses, and yet, at the same time, I noticed his unease to be in the middle of an impersonal machinery whose wheels were turning in his name and by his authority.

Aniline dyes let Ehrlich understand more about the constituents of blood than anyone before him. An array of different cell types, previously unknown, appeared as he stained blood with these coal tar derivatives. They appeared in blushes of pinks and blues and greens, cells and structures gleaming into being. This was the work that led him to find the mast cells his admirer recommended he be rewarded for. They were white cells that existed plentifully in everyone's blood; without dyes, no one had understood them to be different from the other white cells around them.

In St Petersburg, in 1891, Yuri Romanovsky took blood from patients suffering from malaria and stained it. In patients treated with quinine, the malarial parasites were clearly damaged, the first definite indication that the drug acted by attacking the invader rather than supporting the host's defences. The same year Ehrlich, knowing that methylene blue stained the malarial *plasmodium*, gave capsules of the dye to two patients suffering from malaria in Berlin. Both recovered. Unable to deliberately infect animals with malaria, and busy with a project on diphtheria, he never followed the finding up.

From 1896 Ehrlich won his independence. His Institute of Serum Research and Examination was opened in Berlin. Three years later, in 1899, it moved to Frankfurt and was renamed the Royal Prussian Institute for Experimental Therapy. Ehrlich's collaboration with the dye companies continued. They sent him samples of the new colours they produced, and he tried to turn them to new uses.

9 Medical Missionaries

While Germany remained the homeland of the microbe hunters, other nations still played parts. With their large overseas empire, the British were particularly interested in tropical diseases. Men like David Livingstone needed to understand them in order to survive, and wanted to understand them in order to help.

Livingstone's medical investigations went hand in hand with his efforts in quite different forms of exploration. Born in Scotland in 1813, Livingstone grew up as one of seven children all sharing a tenement room with their parents. The room was owned by the mill company where David's father worked, and where David, from the age of ten, went to join him. His education continued, however, at school in the evenings, and in private study by himself or with Dad. By the age of twenty-three Livingstone had saved enough money to put himself through medical school – and simultaneously train as a missionary. Religion and science, he felt, were complementary, the one as much the work of God as the other. In 1840, aged twenty-seven, he qualified for both.

A poor preacher, Livingstone turned out to be a superb missionary, at least in part due to his humility. Rather than trumpeting his message to people whether they were interested or not, Livingstone was content to begin by observation and exploration. 'Christianity, Commerce and Civilisation' is the motto inscribed on his statue at Victoria Falls. It sounds flat and even foolish today, but for Livingstone, it was vivid and real. It meant salvation, through building communities and communication. Medicine was vital to this cause. It was a way of winning friends as well as bringing aid, and it was also essential for survival. European exploration of Africa was limited as much by disease as by the difficulties of diplomacy. From his 1865 *Narrative of an Expedition to the Zambesi*, here are Livingstone's instructions for surviving malaria:

> A remedy composed of from six to eight grains of resin of jalap, the same of rhubarb, and three each of calomel and quinine, made up into four pills, with tincture of cardamoms, usually relieved all the symptoms in five or six hours . . . Quinine after or during the operation of the pills, in large doses every two or three hours, until deafness or cinchonism ensued, completed the cure. The only cases in which we found ourselves completely helpless, were those in which obstinate vomiting ensued.

Livingstone's dosages of quinine were generous enough to make him more successful than his peers, but he, his wife and his daughter eventually died of malaria all the same. The combination of so many different ingredients, in his description from 1865, was a reminder of the extent to which the chemists had not yet revolutionised therapies. The only one that helped was quinine. The others, added to produce diarrhoea, harmed.

Earlier, in a letter dated 22 March 1858, and published on 1 May, Livingstone wrote to the *British Medical Journal*. From the steamer *Pearl*, off the Senegalese coast, he apologised for having been too busy to previously tell the journal's correspondent that 'the employment of arsenic in the disease which follows the bite of the tsetse occurred to my own mind'. He meant that it had occurred to him to

97

use arsenic for a disease that seemed similar to malaria, but impervious to quinine. It was called 'nagana'. Livingstone described an opportunistic animal experiment on a mare bitten repeatedly by tsetse flies, then left to die when it became sick. 'I gave it two grains of arsenic in a little barley daily for about a week,' Livingstone reported, and 'the animal's coat became so smooth and glossy that I imagined I had cured the complaint'.

Despite this early sign of hope, the horse never fully recovered, relapsing some months later:

> I tried the arsenic again; but the mare became like a skeleton, and refused to touch the barley. When I tried to coax her, she turned her mild eye so imploringly, and so evidently meaning, 'My dear fellow, I would rather die of the disease than of the doctor,' that I could not force her.

The horse died six months after her original illness, long enough for Livingstone to feel convinced that the arsenic had helped prolong her life.

The arsenic solution he subsequently recommended was not new. It had been used in England since 1786, not to treat any particular disease but as an all-purpose tonic. There it slowly damaged or killed all those who took it, mistakenly succumbing to its description as being helpful for fevers, malaria, headaches and a host of other conditions for which it did no good at all. (Amongst its other effects, the arsenic destroyed the small blood vessels of the face. The resulting damage gave people's cheeks what was believed to be a healthy glow).

Livingstone's observation of the curative effects of arsenic fell into the grand scheme of similar medical intuitions: more full of optimism than truth. The mare who refused his medicated barley probably made a wise choice, dying more comfortably of the disease than she might have done of the arsenic medicine. It was true that arsenic killed the parasites that caused the disease, but it did the same to horses and to humans.

In the 1890s David Bruce, Australian-born but Scottish-raised, wanted to be a professional sportsman. Instead, a crippling bout of teenage pneumonia sent him towards medicine. Marrying the daughter of a colleague, and a woman who shared his scientific interests, Bruce joined the Army Medical Corps. A posting in Malta gave the couple an opportunity to pursue the methods of their joint hero, Koch. They looked for the cause of an unusual local disease, Malta fever, that affected cattle and sheep and humans. By staining infected blood with the aniline dye gentian violet, they found it.

After a period of research in Koch's own laboratory, the couple were posted to Africa. Asked to investigate an outbreak of nagana, they travelled to what was then Zululand. Nagana was decimating the cattle that the Zulus relied on, but it affected other animals too. David Bruce described it:

> The horse stares, he has a watery discharge from his eyes and nose . . . During this time the animal is becoming more and more emaciated, he looks dull and hangs his head, his coat becoming harsh and thin in places . . . In severe stages, a horse presents a miserable appearance. He is a mere scarecrow, covered by rough hair, which falls off in places . . . At last he falls to the ground and dies of exhaustion.

The Bruces, using the staining techniques they had spent so long learning, found a worm-like parasite in the blood of the affected animals. They showed that it was responsible for the disease, and was spread by the bite of the tsetse fly. In honour of them it was given the name *Trypanosoma brucei*.

Sleeping sickness – the 'African lethargy' – had been known about in Europe from the fourteenth century. During the latter part of the nineteenth, it was spreading. In 1876 a French surgeon reported that it was emptying entire villages in Senegal; twenty years later it was decimating the human population around Lake Victoria. Contemporary estimates there suggested three quarters of a million dead. Together with an Italian, Count Aldo Castellani, the Bruces found a similar organism in the blood of those infected. Sleeping sickness and nagana were extensions of the same disease, both spread by the bite of the inch-long tsetse fly. Arsenic was poisonous to humans. The Bruces showed that it killed trypanosomes too.*

By 1901, researchers at the Pasteur Institute in France were able to use the trypanosome to deliberately infect laboratory rats and mice. That at least opened the way to test putative therapies more easily.

Ehrlich had shown that dyes could selectively stain certain bacteria. He theorised that there were receptors on the surface of bacteria different from those on human cells, and that if poisons gained access through these then they would kill the bacteria without killing the person who carried them. Stains provided a mentally and visually beautiful way of attempting to derive therapies of boundless benefit. 'Initially, therefore,' remembered Ehrlich, 'chemotherapy was a "chromotherapy".' Chemotherapy – the use of chemistry to heal people – was a word that Ehrlich coined. No one better deserved to.

The problem now was how to move forward from a conceptual breakthrough – drugs that could theoretically target bacteria – to finding a practical demonstration. Some stains killed the creatures they were injected into, others accurately coloured only the infective organisms and yet were wholly harmless. If the toxicity could be tied into the selectiveness, the world would become a different place.

* The couple died in 1931, within a few days of each other. 'If any notice is taken of my scientific work when I am gone,' said David on his deathbed, 'I should like it to be known that Mary is entitled to as much of the credit as I am.'

Vereinigte Chemische Werke, a German chemical company, started selling a new arsenic-based treatment for sleeping sickness at the beginning of the twentieth century. The compound had first been made in 1863, but nothing much had ever come of it. Now the Vereinigte chemical works thought it had potential. Without evidence, they sold it on the basis that it was as effective as previous drugs, but massively less toxic. They called it Atoxyl, to drive the message home. There were links between the chemical company and Ehrlich, and it was probably through them that a sample of the drug reached him. He tried it out on trypanosomes and, finding it useless, put it aside and turned to other things.

Then, in 1905, Ehrlich read an English paper suggesting Atoxyl really was active against sleeping sickness. Checking his work, he discovered they were correct. His mistake had been to try the drug out on the isolated organism, the trypanosome. In those circumstances it continued to show no effects. When it was given to a living creature already infected, the story was different. The Pasteur Institute's techniques for infecting mice with sleeping sickness allowed him to see that something strange was happening. Testing his arsenic preparations on isolated trypanosomes, Ehrlich found they still had no impact – but giving them to living animals definitely did. The biological activity of trial compounds, he realised, could only be assessed *in vivo*, not *in vitro*. Life, not glass, was the tool required.

Still, though, the trouble was that the drug lacked sufficient selectivity to be safe. It damaged the infecting organism, but it did so at unacceptable expense, causing blindness and other problems. Atoxyl was badly named, and the claims for its safety that the Vereinigte company made were mistaken. Ehrlich showed that others had muddled the structural nature of the molecule. With a more accurate model, he wondered about the possibility of altering Atoxyl's structure and therefore its effects. Could the selectivity of the molecule be somehow increased, keeping it active against sleeping sickness while making it safer to the humans who suffered from the disease? 'We must strike the parasites and the parasites only, if possible,' said Ehrlich, 'and to do this, we must learn to aim with chemical substances!'

Ehrlich wanted something with a high 'therapeutic index', as toxic as possible for the parasite and as safe as conceivable for the host. In return for funding his research, he agreed to offer any patent rights to the nearby Cassella Dye Works. Deliberately infecting mice with sleeping sickness, Ehrlich tried out over a hundred different dyes to see if he could find any that were toxic to the *Trypanosoma* that caused the disease. Nagana Red became the name of the only one that seemed to work, wiping out the trypanosomes from the blood of the mice. It worked, though, for only a short time. Rather than dying after three or four days, the mice lived for five or six. Ehrlich asked his contacts at the Cassella Dye Works, soon to become part of Hoechst, to prepare him a modified version of the dye. He persuaded them to alter it, suggesting that a modification could make the dye better absorbed by the animals, thereby increasing its therapeutic power. The resulting dye, Trypan Red, was, as he expected, more powerful. Enthusiasm and desperation led to its use in humans. Again, it was not selective enough: it killed trypanosomes well enough, but it killed people too.

In 1905, while he was still continuing with his efforts to develop a drug for sleeping sickness, the cause of syphilis was uncovered. *Treponema pallidum* was the latest germ to be exposed by the new techniques of staining. It took up colour poorly and even with the brightest stains kept a pallid look. Despite that, it appeared a similar organism in many ways to the trypanosomes. Every compound that Ehrlich had produced was fetched out again, and tested for potency against this other disease. Sleeping sickness was important, but it was not much of a problem for the developed world. Syphilis was altogether different.

At first the work went slowly, the only animal model for syphilis being apes, and work with them being laborious and time-consuming. In 1909, though, the biologist Sacachiro Hata arrived from Tokyo to work with Ehrlich. Hata found a way of infecting rabbits with syphilis, making the work quicker and more practical. Testing the 606th of Ehrlich's existing preparations, one that had been abandoned two years earlier as useless against sleeping sickness, Hata found that it worked for syphilis.

Ehrlich insisted on extensive animal experiments to make sure that compound 606 – or Salvarsan, as it came to be called – was free enough of toxicity to do more good than harm. He spoke about magic bullets, but he wanted to be sure he had not produced something more like buckshot, damaging everything around it. Finally convinced that he had not, from 1910 Ehrlich released samples widely, in return for full case information on every patient treated. Syphilis was sexually transmitted, chronic, incurable and eventually fatal. It held a position a hundred years ago roughly equivalent to that of AIDS before the development of the anti-retrovirals that keep that disease at bay. In syphilitics whose infections reached their brains and spinal cords, producing a condition called General Paralysis of the Insane, the effect of Salvarsan was unmistakably miraculous. (A related compound, developed a few years later specifically for trypanosomiasis, was similarly effective for that disease.)

Ehrlich showed that the molecular structure of a drug determined its effects, and he developed the concept of the cell surface receptor, the means by which compounds were selective for certain targets. For all that, Salvarsan was a wonderfully clear indication of science's *inability* to accurately predict a drug's effect without experimentation. As with Atoxyl, culture dishes were not enough. The breakthrough had required rabbits, and lots of them.

103

Sometime later, the Zionist and chemist Chaim Weizmann met Ehrlich, wanting to enrol his support for the proposed Hebrew University in Jerusalem:

I have retained an ineradicable impression of Ehrlich. His figure was small and stocky, but he had a head of great beauty, delicately chiselled; and out of his face looked a pair of eyes which were the most penetrating that I have ever seen – but they were eyes filled with human kindness. Ehrlich knew that I was a chemist, but he did not know what I was coming to see him about. He therefore plunged at once into the subject of his researches. He introduced me to some of his assistants (since become famous) and especially to his rabbits and guinea pigs.

The animals were valuable in themselves, for their colour and their character. And beyond that they were keys to opening up the world, and discovering ways of making it better. Ehrlich loved them.

*

It was not only in Germany and Britain that the aniline dye industry flourished. The New World was getting involved as well. The bays and harbours around New York, once famously full of oysters, wild-life and natural beauty, were becoming polluted and lifeless. In the 1880s, residents of Brooklyn noticed the effects of the blossoming dye industry on the Gowanus Canal, a channel reaching in from the bay. They 'complained of the smell but were more struck by the colours. Dye manufacturers turned the waterway a different pigment every day. The canal was nicknamed "Lavender Lake".'

Odd health beliefs about the industry were not confined to people whose minds exaggerated the fears. For all those who believed without proof that everything which came from industrial processes was unhealthy, there were others who believed the opposite for as little reason. Brooklynites took their asthmatic children to the waters of Lavender Lake, standing them on its bridges in the belief that the rising fumes must have healing powers.

The fallacy common to both groups of people – those who saw only harms, and those who saw only benefits – was ascribing a global value to something that was perfectly ambivalent in itself, and full of variation in its different manifestations. Two German chemists, Fritz Haber (who worked with Bunsen at Heidelberg and with Hofmann in Berlin) and Carl Bosch, spent years at the end of the nineteenth century and the start of the twentieth developing a technique for making ammonia. It meant that people could manufacture fertiliser, increasing the bounty of their land and saving themselves from starvation. The first use of the Haber–Bosch process was not to prevent famine but to worsen the slaughter of the First World War: ammonia was essential for explosives, and as early as 1914 Germany was running out. Haber helped keep the war going another four years, and while it progressed he worked on chemical weapons, and oversaw the first successful use of chlorine gas on the Western Front. His wife, objecting to such horrors, shot herself in the heart.

Organic chemistry, like medicine, offered both therapies and injuries. The difficulty was in telling the difference, and making the choice.

10 Aspirin and Drug Development

The Reverend Stone's discovery of the uses of willow bark in the eighteenth century made it rapidly popular. It was much cheaper than quinine, and widely used as a result. In 1826 the Frenchman Henri Leroux had the first partial success in isolating what seemed to be the active ingredient. Johann Buchner in Munich succeeded in purifying it two years later and first used the name 'salicin' for the concentrated drug. Others found similar methods for the same process. Salicin turned out to be converted by the body into salicylic acid, which was itself generated directly from willow bark by the Italian chemist Raffaele Piria in 1838.

Both salicin and salicylic acid, though, had nasty side effects. They damaged people's guts, causing bleeding, diarrhoea and death. In 1853 a French pharmacist, Charles Gerhardt, figured out a way of buffering the salicylic acid and making it less corrosive. His interests were chemical rather than commercial and, satisfied with his success, he pursued it no further. Several German chemists repeated and improved on Gerhardt's work, also without seeing that it had practical medical potential.

Increases in European population during the nineteenth century meant that malaria grew less common. Swamps and marshes were drained so the land could be farmed. That meant less malaria, which was good, but it also helped to prolong people's confusion about the difference between quinine and willow. Fewer cases of malaria meant less research into the disease, and a continuing delay in appreciating the difference between eliminating a fever and curing a disease.

Rheumatoid arthritis was another condition that, like malaria, seemed to doctors to respond particularly well to extracts of salicin and salicylic acid. Painful swelling of the joints, often accompanied by fever, were the main symptoms of the disease. A Scottish doctor, Thomas Maclagan, wrote to the *Lancet* in 1876 about his experiences in using salicin for the disease. Others later argued over whether he, or a group of German physicians, first stumbled on the treatment. More important is some of the language that Maclagan used. He was initially complacent about the treatment's side effects ('I have never found the least inconvenience follow its use') but encouragingly thoughtful in maintaining some doubts. 'I shall be greatly obliged if those who try the remedy, and do not care to publish their observations,' he wrote, 'would kindly forward to me the results of their experience, be it favourable or otherwise.' The notion that unsuccessful uses of the drug were less likely to get published was implicit. Some progress was being made, both in the capacity of doctors to think and also in their ability to prescribe drugs with at least some benefits.

At the University of Munich, chemists continued to try to do what Perkin had so completely failed in doing – producing synthetic quinine. By 1882 Ernst Otto Fischer, and Wilhelm Koenigs, supervised by Ernst's cousin Emil Fischer, produced novel compounds that they thought were similar to quinine. Although their ideas about quinine's molecular structure later turned out to be mistaken, one of the new molecules they produced did indeed seem to share with quinine the ability to bring down fevers.

The Munich chemists took out a patent and sought a company to back them. They chose a dyestuff manufacturer. The Frankfurt company Farbwerke, vorm. Meister, Lucius & Brüning, had never made a drug before. No dyestuff company ever had. They knew enough about chemicals and markets, however, to spot an opportunity. In 1882, selling their anti-fever drug under the trade name Kairin, from the Greek word for 'timely', they went into this new business. By the following year the company formally created a pharmaceutical division, and soon it became so successful that it needed a simpler name. It became Farbwerke Hoechst, or, in practice, just Hoechst.*

Hoechst's new product was the start, not only of dyestuff companies getting heavily involved in drug manufacture, but also of a range of medications for fevers. Seeing Hoechst's production of Kairin, which was soon attracting bad publicity for the drug's toxic side effects, a group of independent chemists offered Hoechst their alternative drug. It was called Antipyrine, and was introduced on the basis of what the chemists knew about it, which was not a great deal. As with the group that developed Kairin, there were basic mistakes about this drug's structure. Both were largely based on two benzene rings. The first was a tetrahydroquinoline – as quinine was also incorrectly thought to be – and the second was believed to be a tetrahydroquinoline but turned out later, in fact, to be a derivative of pyrazolone, an unrelated molecule. Since a drug's overall effects can even now be predicted only poorly on the basis of its function, these mistakes were less serious than they seemed. The key error was that only a few unstructured tests were performed on animals, and a handful of test doses of each drug given to small numbers of healthy and febrile people. The idea that drugs might do harms, subtler and harder to see than their ability to reduce a fever, did not readily occur to people. 'Among the many remedies that have been discovered to alleviate the ills of suffering humanity,' said the *New York Times* on the first day of 1886, without much evidence, 'none is more important than Antipyrine.' The paper endorsed its safety without

---

* Today, following various changes and mergers, it is a drug company called Sanofi-Aventis, with yearly sales in 2006 worth over 28 billion euros.

justification, but added an important caveat. 'It should be understood that Antipyrine does not claim to cure a disease, it simply reduces temperature.'

Hoechst showed some initial caution in using the drug. After the pre-release tests, they sent it only to hospitals willing to report back on how it performed. By 1884 there were more than forty academic papers, and the majority were positive. For everyone involved in the drug, that felt like enough.

Naphthalene, a coal tar derivative, is poisonous to humans. Not terrifically: it makes up the main ingredient of mothballs, and you need dedication to eat enough of them to kill yourself. Swallow enough mothballs, however, and your red blood cells begin to split apart. Doctors at the University of Strasbourg in the 1880s had no way of knowing this when they started giving naphthalene to patients suffering from worm infestations. Their ignorance of its full effects sounds like a reasonable excuse for their actions; in the context of their time it is usually accepted as being so. Animal experimentation, however, had already been shown to be useful at spotting unexpected toxicity. The willingness of doctors to try novel treatments on their patients, rather than on rabbits, should still grate. It was possible to test extensively for drug safety in animals by the end of the nineteenth century, but few doctors or chemists did.

When Adolf Kussmaul, the head of Strasbourg University's medical department, asked two of his juniors, Arnold Cahn and Paul Hepp, to try out naphthalene's effects on patients with worms, they did so. There appeared to be neither obvious benefits nor harms. Consumed with optimism, and the spirit of haphazard trial and error, they gave it to a patient suffering from a fever rather than from worms. The fever vanished. Publicly, they attributed their discovery of the drug's effect to 'a fortunate accident', a curious euphemism for their willingness to take chances with other people's health.

Naphthalene, however, was meant to smell, just as mothballs do. The drug that successfully treated the patient's fever did not. Cahn and Hepp discovered that what the hospital pharmacy had labelled as naphthalene was not naphthalene at all. They contacted the dye works that had made the product, Kalle & Co., wanting to know what they had got hold of. The drug turned out to be acetanilide, a sweet-tasting, white-coloured derivative of aniline. The company learnt from Cahn and Hepp that they possessed a potential product. But it was a tricky one to sell. Acetanilide was a common compound, meaning there was no way they could secure a patent on it. The solution seemed to be to give it a different name – Antifebrin – and to hope that made it smell a little sweeter. Remarkably, it worked. The branding was enough. Doctors preferred 'Antifebrin' to the cheaper 'acetanilide', and were happy enough to prescribe it by its expensive trade name, even knowing exactly what it was.

In 1889, when an influenza epidemic hit Europe, the habit of taking a drug to banish a fever became cemented in Western culture. Thanks to companies like Kalle and Hoechst, almost everyone could afford to take something. Whether it affected their chances of survival, for better or for worse, was not a question that was seriously addressed. They liked it, their doctors liked it, the drug companies liked it – everyone was happy. The drugs made people feel better, therefore they believed they must be doing them good.

In 1896, Hoechst began selling a slightly adjusted version of Antipyrin under the name Pyramidon. It was three times as powerful – which sounded good, even if the only actual difference it made was that you needed to swallow less of it to achieve the same effect. Like Antipyrin, it became a bestseller. By 1908, Hoechst were doing very well indeed. Since the company making Antifebrin was also doing well, Hoechst bought them. Life looked promising for those making pharmaceuticals.

*

Friedrich Bayer was born in 1825 near Cologne. His father was a silk worker, and at the age of fourteen Bayer began an apprenticeship with a dyestuffs dealership. William Perkin's discoveries were years ahead, so the dyes they used came from animals and vegetables rather than aniline.*

Bayer was successful, setting himself up in business and trading dyes across Europe. He met a like-minded fellow named Johann Weskott, and the two men joined forces. Perkin's innovations were sweeping across their business, and they needed to respond. They imported some of the early aniline dyes and tried to understand how to produce them themselves. In 1863 they founded the firm of Friedrich Bayer & Co.

It grew steadily, and when Bayer died in 1880, and Weskott in 1881, it employed over 300 people. Weskott's and Bayer's descendants inherited the company. They renamed it (not with notable linguistic flair) as Farbenfabriken vormals Friedrich Bayer & Company – 'the Dye Factory formerly known as Friedrich Bayer & Company' – and raised money by a sell-off of shares. Part of their purpose was to invest more capital in research, which meant paying for laboratories and for chemists to fill them.

* In that sense, they were natural, but dyes always involved a degree of artifice. Roots were grubbed up, shellfish gathered, juices extracted, cloths soaked. The chemical reactions of mud and vinegar, madder and indigo and cochineal, were managed by people without much aid from machines. The coal tar industry extracted colour, not from plants, but from the ancient remains of plants, and it used many machines. But natural dyes still needed the interventions of the dye makers, and factory-made ones could still be safer than naturally occurring ones containing lead or arsenic. The catastrophic history of medicine is partly the result of ascribing qualities without reasonable evidence, and one way of doing that is to think of natural as being good and artificial as being bad. In 1999 the *Lancet* told the story of a twenty-five-year old man found comatose in a Berlin park. His heart stopped for over seven hours, his circulation kept going all that time by chest compressions. While others did what they could for him, a nurse going through his pockets for clues about his collapse found bits of yew tree. Remarkably, the man regained consciousness and survived. He often ate plants, he explained on waking, 'since natural foods were "healthy"'.

One of the new chemists was named Carl Duisberg. On his twenty-third birthday, having previously struggled to scratch a living with his chemistry qualifications, Duisberg became a full-time Bayer employee. Within a short space of time he developed new ways of arriving at two existing colours (thereby circumventing patent law) and discovered a third colour that was entirely new – to the productions of organic chemists, at least. He was rapidly promoted. From being handed research projects became able to give ones of his own devising to other staff.

Reading the descriptions of Antifebrin in 1885, Duisberg realised that this was something Bayer should be competing with. He had the company produce slightly altered versions of the compound. One seemed to work well, and the following year Bayer put Phenacetin onto the open market. It sold prodigiously, but Duisberg continued directing the company to try to develop alternatives. By 1890 he was largely in control of Bayer. In 1893, in collaboration with an eminent physician named Joseph von Mering, Duisberg and Bayer tried out a compound structurally similar to Phenacetin. N-(4-hydroxyphenyl)ethanamide was soon renamed Paracetamol, but just as quickly rejected. It worked well, concluded von Mering, but it was toxic to the blood. Paracetamol was shelved as useless.

Meanwhile, Hoechst's Antipyrine was selling well. It took until 1934 for doctors to notice that Antipyrine killed people. Not many, but some. Their realisation did not come as the result of a careful trial, comparing those who took it with those who did not. Instead it came because the blood disorder it caused was rare enough to get attention. In contrast it took until 1948 for people to notice the toxicity of Antifebrin. The liver and kidney damage it caused was far less remarkable. Not that it did less harm, it was just that slow failure of liver and kidneys was relatively common, so without structured trials capable of recognising the cause of these extra deaths, it took longer for anyone to connect them with the drug. The same was true for Phenacetin, discovered in the 1880s, where concerns over kidney damage took the best part of a century to surface. In 1949 a group of American researchers reported their discovery that the body turned Phenacetin into two different compounds. One, phenetidine, was responsible for most of the toxicity, the other, which was actually Paracetamol, for most of the benefits.

Paracetamol's rediscovery in this manner prompted a revision of von Mering's opinion that it was too dangerous to use. Most of the explanations for its peculiar rejection in the 1890s suggest that there were impurities in the compound that von Mering tested, which accounted for his mistaken conclusion. His eminence kept anyone from noticing this for another fifty years.

*

In the late nineteenth century coal tar, along with its derivative phenol, was being used as an external antiseptic. Observations that the two compounds prevented decay in meat and vegetables led on to their application to human wounds. On that basis the Scottish surgeon Lister developed antisepsis – which, developed by extension into asepsis, revolutionised surgery. Antisepsis meant deploying compounds that were toxic to the micro-organisms causing infectious diseases; asepsis meant keeping operating theatres and surgical wounds so scrupulously clean that the bugs never got a chance to establish themselves in the first place. Not only was Lister able to make theatres safer places to be than ever before, enabling surgeons to open up chests and skulls and abdomens with every hope that their patients would survive, he also used numbers to demonstrate the power of his new techniques effectively, comparing survival percentages before and after his technique's introduction. The gradual increase of statistics in medicine was subtler than that of asepsis, but every bit as powerful.

By the 1870s, doctors had realised that phenol and coal were too corrosive to be useful wound dressings, and certainly too toxic to take internally. Their potential, however, was something these doctors were very interested in. They were learning about the impact of bacteria on the outside of the body, and speculating about their influence within. Disinfecting the gut seemed to hold out therapeutic promise. Getting people to swallow phenol was similar to having them swill down bleach – it killed the germs well enough, but the overall effect on the patient was not good. It was too corrosive to the guts. Salicylic acid become popular as an alternative. It was antiseptic and, although it was still caustic, it was mild in comparison with phenol. In 1853 the German chemist Hermann Kolbe figured out how to make salicylic acid directly from coal tar, without having to trouble with the willow.* From 1874 the process was successfully industrialised, and salicylic acid became very much cheaper as a result.

By 1897, Bayer chemists had developed versions of salicylic acid that they hoped would provide all the benefits with fewer of the harms. Salicylic acid could irritate the stomach lining to the point of dissolving a hole in it. One of the alternative versions that Bayer investigated, acetylsalicylic acid, was the buffered compound previously made by the French academic chemist Charles Gerhardt in 1853. Gerhardt had done nothing with his discovery besides publishing it.

Bayer employees showed great interest in the substance, until a leading member of the company, Heinrich Dreser, rejected it as being damaging to the heart. His colleague, Arthur Eichengrün, thought he was wrong. Eichengrün pushed for clinical experiments, but was overruled. Ignoring this, he arranged for acetylsalicylic acid to be secretly tested by doctors in Berlin. The image of evil drug company employees, risking the lives of helpless patients, is not appropriate. Eichengrün shared his generation's complacency about

---

* Or with meadowsweet, which was the alternative plant source for salicin and salicylic acid. The German chemist Karl Lowig had shown this in 1835.

the long-term risk of drugs, and its mistaken optimism in the power of chemists to correctly predict effects on the human body, but his ignorance was sincere rather than manipulative. Before having the drug tested on Berlin patients, Eichengrün tried it out on himself.

The drug performed better in Berlin than even Eichengrün expected. It eased fevers as well as the symptoms of rheumatoid arthritis, and it seemed to have fewer side effects than either salicin or salicylic acid. Given that Eichengrün had tested the drug behind Dreser's back, it was unsurprising that the latter took against it. The news of the drug's benefits came from independent doctors, but when the reports reached Dreser, he decided that his own prejudices were more reliable. 'This is the usual Berlin boasting,' Dreser wrote on the report, 'the product has no value.'

Carl Duisberg settled the argument by ordering a second study done. When it supported Eichengrün, he put Bayer's weight behind the product. Since the product had been created by acetylation, and one of the sources for salicin had originally been not just willow but also meadowsweet – *Spirea ulmaria* – Eichengrün put an 'a' in front of 'spirea', jiggled the letters around a little, and came up with the new drug's trade name: Aspirin.

The first account of Aspirin's development by Bayer was published in 1933, the year after the Nazi Party came to power. Eichengrün, being Jewish, was not mentioned.

11   Cough Medicine Called Heroin

Bayer invested heavily in research, and in ways of making that research as good as possible. The company spent huge amounts on well-equipped laboratories and carefully designed programmes of animal testing. They supported their scientists generously, and encouraged individuals to specialise in either drug development or testing. A dyestuff company had first released a medication in 1882 – Hoechst and Kairin – yet within a decade Bayer and its competitors were orienting themselves in a new, recognisably modern way towards the research and production of novel pharmaceuticals.

Adapting existing medications was an attractive way to begin. Often that meant finding ways to produce the same drugs in a different manner, circumventing a competitor's patent just as Duisberg had done with dyes at the beginning of his commercial career. Actually amending compounds, in order to make them safer or more powerful, was an alternative way forwards. While Bayer continued to improve upon the willow, and continued to fail in synthesising quinine, it also looked elsewhere. With few effective drugs in the world, it was no surprise that they quickly turned their attention to the poppy.

Since the isolation of morphine by Friedrich Wilhelm Sertürner in 1805, chemists had been tinkering with it – often more out of curiosity than with any more purposeful intent. In Scotland and London a few modifications had been made. Some of these helped develop chemical theories, establishing ideas about the way different molecular structures gave rise to particular effects.

In 1874 at St Mary's Hospital in London, Charles Alder Wright developed a new compound, diacetylmorphine, and sent it to F. M. Pierce in Manchester for testing on dogs and rabbits. A thousand years before, Rhazes in Baghdad had written on the importance of comparisons, trying to distinguish the effects of his therapy for meningitis by applying it to some patients and not others, and then comparing them. The degree to which these ideas had escaped medical thought for ten centuries was clear in Wright's approach: although his knowledge of chemistry was far more accurate than that of tenth-century Persia, he used no control animals. As a result, he was left with no clear idea of what diacetylmorphine did and showed no further interest in it.

Carl Duisberg's Bayer, meanwhile, were looking for ways of improving opium. The alkaloid codeine was isolated from the poppy in 1832. It showed some of the same power as morphine to suppress irritating coughs, and at the same time it had a much milder effect on the mind. This drew the interest of Bayer chemists who were seeking drugs that were gentler than the all-powerful morphine. They knew that adding acetyl groups to other compounds had produced exactly those effects, softening them and making them more useful. Felix Hoffmann was the Bayer chemist who acetylated salicylic acid on 10 August 1897 to produce Aspirin. Within two weeks he also acetylated morphine.

Joseph von Mering, the doctor who had advised Bayer in 1893 that Paracetamol was not worth developing, was working for Merck by 1897. Starting in an apothecary's shop in Darmstadt, in the south-west of Germany, what began as a family business in 1668 had continued in the same vein. From the early years of the nineteenth century Emanuel Merck, inheriting the family business, began to expand it. Unlike most of his competitors, he was in charge of a company whose interest in drugs pre-dated the work of William Perkin and his aniline dyes. Merck asked von Mering to test the acetylated version of morphine and give his opinion. Von Mering was unimpressed, and suggested Merck ignore it.

Hofmann's acetylated morphine – diacetylmorphine or simply diamorphine – was tested with more interest by Bayer, who gave it to animals and found that their breathing became deeper and slower. In a world plagued by tuberculosis, with its chronic breathlessness and cough, this looked promising. Bayer staff tried it on themselves. It worked, they found, tremendously. Coughs vanished. People who took it felt strong and wonderful and pain-free. In fact, they felt heroic. From September 1898, Bayer began marketing their new drug for relief of the symptoms of respiratory illnesses. They called it Heroin.

It sold rapidly. Early studies showed no evidence of its being addictive. It was, of course, but the studies were too poorly designed to pick that up. But it was not so immediately addictive that the first doctors and patients who used it noticed this for themselves.* Bayer chemists were confident, on the basis of what they knew of the drug's structure, that addiction would not be a problem. So they never designed tests capable of proving their prejudices wrong. The powers of chemists and doctors were increasing and success was not the sort of thing to encourage humility.

It required no methodical powers of observation to see that Heroin got rid of coughs, eased pains and generally made people feel better. Often they felt a lot better, even if they had been feeling pretty good to begin with. Ideas that Heroin helped people breathe were the first ones to change. It became apparent that Heroin's effects on breathing were exactly those of morphine, and of laudanum and opium before it. By the time it was eventually discovered that

---

* 'You don't wake up one morning and decide to be a drug addict,' wrote the novelist William Burroughs. 'It takes at least three months' shooting twice a day to get any habit at all.'

Heroin's main action was the result of the body simply converting it into morphine, people had already noticed enough of the similarities not to be surprised. Heroin confirmed that even the world's best chemists and doctors, acting on the knowledge of a drug's structure, could not necessarily predict its effects ahead of time. It was not a lesson that was widely learnt, or that researchers found easy to remember.

Bayer stopped producing Heroin in 1913. It had become too linked in the public mind with addiction, particularly in America, and the profits did not justify the bad publicity. Other companies carried on making it, and the drug continues to be a useful and effective medication, although some countries, like the USA, ban it even for therapeutic use. For patients with smashed bones, failing hearts, gnawing cancers or suffocating breathlessness, it works very well. Sometimes morphine is all that is available, in which case a larger dose achieves the same effect. Bayer's website, which proudly records the company's production of Aspirin, makes no mention of Heroin. That seems a pity. There are worse things to be ashamed of, and Bayer, as we will see, went on to be involved in many of them.

12   Francis Galton Almost Reforms Medicine

By the end of the nineteenth century, the productions of science were impressive. Methodologies, as well as results, were getting better. Just as some of the approaches that made up chemistry were developed in pursuit of other goals — alchemy and intoxication — so the constituents of scientific method itself often came from unlikely quarters.

'Tall, slim, neatly dressed, with a forehead like the dome of St Paul's', Francis Galton possessed a mind quite remarkable enough to suit the shape of his skull. The origins and capacities of this mind, as well as their possible reflections in the shape of his head, were of great interest to Galton. Hereditary genius and phrenology were two of his interests. So, however, were mathematics, psychology, fingerprints, the weather, whistling, Shakespeare, genetics, African exploration, yawning, the Middle East, twins, families, novels and evolution.

At the age of sixteen, in 1838, Francis Galton was sitting down with his wealthy and intellectually distinguished family. It was 'chilly out of doors, while indoors our family party were assembled in cosy comfort at dessert, after a good dinner, with a brightly burning fire, shining mahogany table, wine, fruits, and all the rest'. A medical career was being discussed for Galton, and a family friend had promised to offer him a taste of it before he committed himself. So it was that a note arrived offering Galton the immediate opportunity for leaving dinner, venturing outside and going to see the post-mortem on a newly dead housemaid. 'Oh,' he exclaimed, 'the mixture of revulsion, wonder, interest, and excitement!'

The girl had died, rather rapidly, from a perforation in her stomach – exactly the sort of thing that willow caused, and that doctors had not yet identified as one of the drug's side effects. As he was sewing up her belly, the surgeon doing the autopsy pricked his finger. Germs from the girl's corpse were inoculated into his flesh, and over the following days the infection grew worse and the surgeon's future looked bleak. Against expectations, he eventually survived.

Impressed by these serious experiences, Galton launched himself into medicine. At the Birmingham General Hospital in the early 1840s he 'learnt the difference between infusions, decoctions, tinctures, and extracts' – all of which, with the exceptions of cinchona, opium and willow, varied on a scale of therapeutic value from poisonous through to useless. Galton availed himself of liquorice (used as a diuretic, a drug to make people urinate) and of poppy seeds. Both tasted pleasant, and neither had any particular effect on him. These were years 'long before those of chloroform, and many long years before that of Pasteur and Sir Joseph Lister. The stethoscope was considered generally to be new-fangled.'

It fell to Galton to deal with the traumas that he could, and to call for help when needed. He set bones, fixed dislocations, staunched bleeding sometimes and created it often – cutting open veins and arteries in the belief that losing blood was good for people. He dressed burns, watching the neat bandages fester with pus as the patients deteriorated. He shaved heads, using the blood from the wounds as a lather, and stitched gaping scalps. And he developed the feeling that there was something to be learnt from 'the apparently unmoral course of Nature', this stream of misery and suffering.

'Blind Nature seems to vivisect ruthlessly,' he wrote. 'Let us as reasonable creatures elicit all the good we can from her vivisections.' The horrors of the patients watching each other die struck him, as did the uselessness of much of what he had to offer. Under orders to apply a mustard dressing to a girl sick with typhus, he heard her plead to be left alone. 'Please leave me in peace,' she begged him. 'I know I am dying, and am not suffering.' Ignoring the instructions from his teacher, Galton did as she asked.

Perhaps because of Galton's heritage – there seemed to be no one in the family who was not a Fellow of the Royal Society, a Darwin, or a gifted scientist – he remained aware of medicine's lacks, even as he was beguiled by its practices. A man became unconscious with drink, and as he lay on the road a wagon rolled over his legs, crushing the bones past hope of recovery. A surgeon amputated both without his waking up, and Galton could not work out why doctors did not deliberately use alcohol to knock their patients senseless before operations. It was a very reasonable question to ask, without any obviously good answer. Another man 'stumbled into a cauldron of scalding pitch'. He was pulled away, but in places the pitch was stuck to his melted skin and could not be removed. One leg was encased with the stuff, and the doctors could do little for it. The other was not so badly damaged, and they dressed it properly with a healing poultice. As the days went by, the more severely injured and more lightly medicated leg recovered much more quickly. 'It seemed clear', concluded Galton, 'that the art of dressing was far behind what was possible.' Despite his insight, he failed to draw the full lesson: that this particular natural vivisection strongly suggested either that dressings made wounds worse or that pitch made them better. Blind belief in the utility of medications was stuck onto people's minds, the way the boiling pitch stuck to flesh, but without any of the wholesome qualities. 'I was so keen at my medical work,' said Galton, 'I began by taking small doses of all that were included in the pharmacopoeia, commencing with the letter A. It was an interesting experience, but had obvious drawbacks.'

It seemed to him that progress was being made. 'The signs of advance were all about and in the air. The microscope had rather suddenly attained a position of much enhanced importance.' This was in 1839, almost two hundred years after Leeuwenhoek had come across his first magnifying glass and gone on to describe microscopic life. The microscope was an impressive piece of technology, but the only thing it helped a doctor to offer was an extra bit of pomp: there were no benefits for the patients.

'There is still much lack of exact knowledge of what Nature can do without assistance from medicine,' wrote Galton shrewdly, 'if aided only by cheering influences, rest, suggestions, and good nursing.' The lack of knowledge was because nobody had yet thought of the right way of seeking for it. Without asking nature the proper questions and in reliable ways, doctors received no useful answers. Galton suggested a way that they might – if they had a mind to – approach the world much more effectively. 'Suppose two different and competing treatments of a particular malady,' he suggested. 'Let the patients suffering under it be given the option of being placed under Dr. A. or Dr. B., the respective representatives of the two methods, and the results be statistically compared. A co-operation without partisanship between many large hospitals ought to speedily settle doubts that now hang unnecessarily long under dispute.' Doctors, however, thought differently. Dr A. could see no reason for such an examination, since it was clear to him that his methods worked. Dr B., for all that he felt Dr A. to be sadly mistaken, was equally sure in his own designs. They disagreed over many things, but were equally sure their own ideas were correct. Neither could see the need for a trial of them.

What follows, in Galton's autobiography, is a passage that can sound a little bland if you read it too quickly. In fact it is a summary of why doctors had always failed their patients, an explanation for why unstructured observations, and a reliance on experience and intuition, are misleading:

> Medical statistics are, however, the least suitable of any I know for refined comparisons, because the conditions that cannot be, or at all events are not taken into account, are local, very influential, and apt to differ greatly. It is, however, humiliating to find how much has failed to attract attention for want of even the rudest statistics. I doubt whether the unaided apprehension of man suffices to distinguish between the frequency of what occurs on an average four times in ten events and one that occurs five times.

In other words, people and their diseases vary so much that using your own personal experience to compare them is generally useless. This man's tuberculosis is not the same as that woman's; this child's sore throat is different from her mother's. The prospect of making accurate comparisons becomes hopeless. Galton is making the point that if you have seen ten episodes of a disease – often spread over a period of time – you are unlikely to notice the difference between an outcome that occurs four times as opposed to five. In other words, if your medicine increases someone's likelihood of living by a quarter – or, similarly, makes them more likely to die – you will not see it. This was why doctors in the seventeenth century had been so slow to notice that cinchona, so brilliant at treating malaria, was better than Peruvian balsam bark, which was useless: many people who got malaria recovered anyway, and many of those given cinchona died all the same. The Jesuit bark made more than a quarter's difference and yet many doctors were unsure if it really helped.

Galton gave examples of the medical errors he could see, of connections overlooked and causes of disease that were misunderstood.

He was particularly struck with the medical habit of declaring, with absolute conviction, for the superiority of particular diets – convictions which varied drastically between doctors. Alcohol was something else that the medical profession always thought it knew the best use for. Galen, acting as physician to the Roman emperor Marcus Aurelius, worked his way through the imperial cellars, searching for the healthiest wines to offer his patient. He was convinced that there was a difference between them. After much research, dutifully undertaken, Galen concluded that the healthiest wine was the one that tasted best. A friend of Galton's, searching through the records of his 'very old and eminent firm of wine merchants', had looked at what doctors prescribed over the years for his company's customers. He found 'that every class of wine had in its turn been favoured by the doctors'. No one, in other words, had the faintest clue. By advocating statistical trials, Galton was suggesting the way in which proper comparisons might help them to try and find out.

As a doctor, Galton never got started. In 1844 his father died. 'Being much upset and craving for a healthier life, I abandoned all thought of becoming a physician.' The world was poorer for it. Partly through his work, however, statistics penetrated a little further into medical thought.

13 Antibiotics and Nazi Nobels

Proof of the possible is exciting, both for inventors and their commercial backers. Now that drugs existed which killed off syphilis and trypanosomes, there was the palpable prospect of making others that destroyed germs of equal or greater menace for human life.

Cassella Dye Works were absorbed with Bayer and other companies into the I. G. Farben conglomerate in 1925. The 'syndicate of dyestuff corporations' – Interessen-Gemeinschaft Farbenindustrie – was a creation masterminded by Carl Duisberg. Impressed by the way American oil companies formed successful cartels, he led Germany's emerging pharmaceutical corporations into doing the same. It helped cut competition, and keep profits high, but it did not put an end to attempts to benefit the consumer. In 1929 I. G. Farben opened an expensive and vastly well-equipped research laboratory. The man in charge was the physician Gerhard Domagk, a student of Ehrlich's.

At the age of nineteen, while still a medical student, Domagk had served in Germany's army on the Western Front. By Christmas of 1914 he was wounded, and spent the rest of the war helping with problems of hygiene. Cholera, typhus and dysentery, as well as medical helplessness in treating them, made deep impressions on him, along with the way in which even aseptic surgery was not enough to prevent horrific infections and gangrene.

Mankind had been worse off before, without even a knowledge of germ theory and the value of cleanliness. Yet an awareness of medical futility, along with great advances in basic sciences, prompted doctors to wonder about how badly they were doing and how much they might improve. It was a healthy impulse, not least for the scepticism and acceptance of ignorance that came with it. With science and technology rapidly advancing in many fields, complacency about medical knowledge looked increasingly old-fashioned. Of the ten million soldiers who died in the First World War, roughly half lost their lives due to infections. Even a minor wound, a scratch, was often enough. That seemed a problem that doctors should be able to do something about.

The commercial benefit of any potential bacteria-killing drug – what today we would call an antibiotic – was as clear as the medical need. I. G. Farben, knowing this, backed its workers well: 'The management of the . . . dye factories always found ways and means of supporting us – who were engaged in scientific research – indeed, they assisted us far more than did the state'. Domagk thought that there was something remarkable about this, that neither 'sickness funds' nor insurance companies, despite their capital and their own financial interests in keeping members healthy, seemed to feel the responsibilities or see the opportunities that drug companies did. A lot of the credit for Farben's enlightened thinking, felt Domagk, was owed to Duisberg.

Since the introduction of Salvarsan in 1910 – Ehrlich's compound number 606 – chemists and doctors had been searching more seriously for compounds able to kill the common bacteria causing human disease. Domagk's innovation was to set up a screening system, one that was both thoughtfully methodical and on an unprecedented scale. A visiting Englishman told of 'enormous laboratories in which they did nothing but take compound after compound and test its ability to deal with infections in animals'. Using these labs, Domagk pursued Ehrlich's inspiration about the selectivity of dyes, and the selective toxicity that might go with them.

By 1890 doctors were well aware that immunity was an important concept in human health. Smallpox, mumps and measles were diseases that you got only once. After that you were either dead or permanently immune – this was what had allowed Edward Jenner to successfully popularise vaccination against smallpox from 1796. The new serum therapy relied on the experimental observation that some degree of immunity could be transferred along with this blood fluid. Emil Behring showed in 1891 that serum taken from an animal already immune to diphtheria could help treat another in the midst of suffering from it. The first human use of serum therapy came that same year, on Christmas Day, on a child in Berlin.

For bacterial infections, attempts at serum therapy were based on injecting animals – usually horses – with the bacterium you wished to attack. Serum from the horse was then injected into a person suffering from that bacterium. Unlike the unmistakable impact of Salvarsan, the effects of these treatments were not always clear. The reaction of the initial animals to bacteria differed, as did the responses of different people to serum from those animals. Added to this, not all bacterial infections were fatal. Many people recovered, regardless of whether they were given serum therapy. And some who were given the serum died as a result, their own bodies reacting violently to it. Many others suffered milder side effects – 'serum sickness' was a constellation of fevers, rashes, joint pains and other problems, sometimes worse than the disease itself. Success and failure, in other words, were difficult for doctors to tell apart.

Our linguistic habit in medicine is to talk about risks versus benefits. It is a hangover from thousands of years of complacency. If you took someone with pneumonia, and gave him or her serum from a prepared horse, it was clear that there were risks. The patient might get serum sickness, and might die. The benefits were equally uncertain. That is, the balance was not between risks and benefits, the balance was between *harms* and benefits. Neither was certain, and any real treatment had a chance – a risk – of doing good just as it had a risk of doing harm. Speaking of 'risks and benefits' too easily makes it seem as though the good things were guaranteed and only the bad ones are difficult to predict.

Methodical efforts to balance harms against benefits profited greatly from the development of serum therapy, clearly dangerous yet clearly useful. There were increasing efforts to design experiments that investigated this uncertainty reliably. These were thought through in a way that the world had never seen before:

> The good results of insulin on patients with diabetes or of liver treatment in pernicious anaemia are so constant that the trial of these remedies in a very few cases was enough to establish their value. With the antiserum treatment of lobar pneumonia the conditions are very different. The action of the serum is only that of a partial factor for good, and its influence may be overwhelmed by an infection that has been allowed several days to establish its dominance in the patient, or by other complicating factors that weaken the patient's resistance. In order to measure precisely what this partial benefit may be it would be necessary to take two groups of cases of identical severity and initial history and compare the sickness and the fatality in each, the one being treated with serum and the other serving as a control. But this is impracticable . . .

The authors, members of the Medical Research Council Therapeutic Trials Committee, were writing in 1934 about their trial of serum therapy. In the *British Medical Journal* they argued that the creation of two such deliberately well-matched groups was impossible. They felt the number of people whose physical conditions were identical was simply too small. Reading their report, it is clear that the real reason was also apparent to them, even if they did not say it explicitly. No matter how much you tried to find cases that were identical, you never could. Even if you took identical twins and infected them at the same moment and with the same bug – an unthinkable experiment – you could not actually guarantee that your two subjects were the same. One twin might be historically weaker then the other, or currently more tired. Even those who were genetically identical still possessed some differences, the result of their environments. It was not that there were too few identical patients, it was that there were actually none whatsoever. It was impossible ever to expect that one patient's situation should be *exactly* that of another.

To get around this, from 1933 a number of British hospitals tried assigning consecutive patients to different approaches. If the first pneumonia patient on the ward got serum therapy, the next would not. In the course of things, they hoped, everything would balance out. The system of alternate allocation did away with any need for doctors to try to 'match' people. It meant that doctors did not need to try to assess every factor they knew of that affected someone's health. Crucially, it meant that it did not even matter if there were important influences that the doctors were completely unaware of. Stick one person into one treatment group, the next into another, and whatever differences there were between them would be ironed out, whether you understood those differences or not. So long, that is, as you took enough people.

This allowance for ignorance and inability was revolutionary. Doctors had always been human, always capable of making mistakes or of not knowing everything there was to know and not seeing everything there was to see. Here, rather than presuming that they could behave perfectly, they built a system that did not require them to. It did not come easily, and some doctors were horrified at the attempt. John Cowan, a Scottish doctor, wrote to the MRC to protest at the trial's methods:

> . . . serum seems to me to be proved to be beneficial . . . It should be available in consequence in ALL hospitals . . . The days of controls are no longer possible: it is not fair to them.

The intuition of doctors, he was arguing, was too reliable to need any external support. Physicians were perfectly capable of telling whether a treatment was working. Withholding a new drug from a group of people, in order to compare what happened to them with what happened to those who were given it, was cruel and unfair.

Enough of the trial doctors felt similarly to compromise its results. Alternate allocation was not robust enough, not in the face of doctors' suspicions that they could tell who would benefit from serum and who would not. Some of those suspicions may not even have been conscious, but that did not matter. The doctors did not manage to stick with the scheme. Alternate allocation meant that doctors knew which treatment a patient would get if entered into the trial. They were able to withhold their sickest and healthiest patients, trying to match them up with the treatment they thought likely to suit them best. They agreed with the principles of doing a trial, but could not get over their feeling that, for some patients, they already knew which treatment was likely to be best.

In the end, different things happened at different hospitals. 'The variation in results at the different centres cannot be explained,' said the report, diplomatically alluding to the fact that the doctors were cheating. Over 1933 and 1934, doctors in Aberdeen, Edinburgh and London managed to study 530 patients with pneumonia. Of these, 241 were given serum therapy. Representing the combined experience of three hospitals and a whole group of doctors, the authors who wrote about the study were still worried that these numbers were too few to tame the play of chance. It was a heartening conclusion, and the complete opposite of John Cowan's belief that his own personal experience, based on watching a vastly smaller number of cases, enabled him to divine exactly the risks of a new therapy.

Serum therapy was cautiously adopted by the British. The trial, published in 1934, suggested the treatment was beneficial for certain patients. Neither the trial's methodology nor its results were marvellous, but the search for antibiotics was proving fruitless, and people were losing interest and hope in it. Many in the medical profession felt that Ehrlich's magic bullets were simply not possible. Using a horse as a living factory to make serum gave the occasional good result, and the odd bad one. Lots of doctors decided it was the best there was.

Streptococcus pyogenes was particularly fatal at the time. It accounted for many deaths from wounds during the First World War, and in the influenza pandemic that followed. At I. G. Farben, Domagk isolated a particular strain of the streptococcus from a dead patient. He grew samples of the bug until he found one that behaved with astonishing consistency. Using mice, Domagk found that they reliably died four days after being injected with the streptococcus.

This sort of repeatability was exactly what the real world of clinical medicine lacked. With a 100 per cent death rate amongst the mice, Domagk knew that any survivors would owe their lives to whatever experimental treatment they received. It gave him an effective way of testing a large number of drugs in a short space of time.

Early experiments confirmed the wisdom of using animals in order to avoid killing humans with experimental drugs. A range of compounds were known to have some antibacterial properties, based on their actions in a culture dish or a test tube. Domagk tried some that were based on gold, a popular therapy. They helped the mice survive the streptococcus, but they killed them in other ways. The gold destroyed healthy kidneys. As a drug, its aim was not precise enough to be a magic bullet. Compounds based on dyes were safer, and in culture dishes they actually worked well, killing bacteria, but in animals they were ineffective.

Using a technique developed to make dyes more colourfast, I. G. Farben's team presented Domagk with a new stain. In December 1932, Domagk tried it out on streptococcus cultures. It had no effect. Domagk took this apparently useless new dye and tried it out on mice all the same. On 20 December, taking twenty-six mice, Domagk injected all of them with a fatal dose of streptococcus. An hour and a half later he gave twelve a dose of the dye. Here was the difference between him and most doctors. John Cowan felt that serum therapy worked so well for pneumonia that 'control' patients were unnecessary, even unethical. That was in a disease where most people got better anyway, and the treatment could kill. Domagk had mice that were virtually guaranteed to die, yet he kept fourteen as controls, just to make sure. The methodological care taken when experimenting with animals had leapt beyond that which was used in humans. Four days later, on Christmas Eve 1932, all of the control mice were dead. All of the ones given the dye were alive.

Prontosil rubrum – the second part of the dye's name referring to its red colour – was kept largely secret for the next three years. Exactly why was never made clear; corporate worries about securing patent protection may have been responsible. On 15 February 1935, Domagk finally published his results.

There was remarkably little excitement, despite no drug having previously worked against this form of overwhelming sepsis that was such a common cause of death worldwide. Perhaps as a result, doctors found it difficult to imagine that any drug *could* work. A widespread disbelief in the possibility of effective antibiotics provoked the prejudice that Domagk's new drug was probably not up to much.

In London, a doctor named Leonard Colebrook was in charge of research at Queen Charlotte's Hospital. It was a maternity hospital, and Colebrook's particular interest was in puerperal fever. The early suggestions, of Oliver Wendell Holmes and others, that puerperal fever was spread from woman to woman by the hands of those who looked after them, had by this time been accepted. Streptococcus was the cause, infecting the wounds left in a woman's genitals after she gave birth. In 1920, a friend of Colebrook's lost his wife to the disease. Moved, Colebrook centred his career on it from then on.

Between 1934 and 1935, Queen Charlotte's Hospital admitted 210 women infected with puerperal fever. Forty-two of them died. That was despite the best efforts of Colebrook and his staff, all of whom understood germ theory and the importance of hygiene in preventing its spread. (For comparison, in 2000 eighty-five British women died during or in the few weeks after giving birth. That was the national total number of maternal deaths, from all causes, in or out of hospital.)

Reading about Domagk's new therapy, and finding it more interesting than his colleagues did, Colebrook asked I. G. Farben to supply him with some Prontosil. From what Colebrook read, the drug seemed impressive, but he was uncertain if its benefits would apply to the women he cared for. Carefully, he began to try to discover if they did.

First of all he tried repeating Domagk's experiments on mice. Colebrook was encouraged, even though the drug did not seem as effective as in Germany. His next step was giving the drug to women already seriously infected with the streptococcus, women so sick that there was little likelihood that even a poisonous drug could make their chances worse. When they appeared to benefit, Colebrook starting giving it to others who were less unwell. Out of a series of thirty-eight women given Prontosil by Colebrook, three died. The case fatality rate for the disease over the previous year had been 20 per cent, forty-two out of 210. With the drug, and aware that he was still tending to select out the sickest of the women, Colebrook was achieving a fatality rate of about 8 per cent.

Despite his excitement, and his desperation to find an effective treatment for puerperal fever, Colebrook was still not sure. 'It behoves us to be very cautious in drawing conclusions', he wrote, 'as to the curative effect of any remedy upon puerperal infections.' The disease was hard to diagnose and hard to predict. Domagk's mice had definitely been infected with streptococcus and they all, reliably, died. Neither the diagnosis nor the outcome was quite so clear among women at Queen Charlotte's.

Adding to the confusion was a remarkable suggestion by scientists at France's Pasteur Institute. Prontosil's effectiveness, they said, was not because it was a dye. Despite the fact that the ability of aniline dyes to stain bacteria had been the trigger for Prontosil's development, they thought there was no relationship between the drug's colour and its actions. The portion that made the chemical red, they argued, was actually irrelevant. What made it work was the other part of it, the remnant left when the dye part of the drug was removed. Chemically this consisted of a sulphone group connected to an amine. It was called sulphanilamide.

This was hugely important. Sulphanilamide had been discovered and described in 1908, the product of a chemist's doctoral studies. Neither I. G. Farben nor anyone else could now patent it. If the Pasteur Institute were correct, not only was their insight relevant for the future development of similar drugs, it also meant that the production and sale of sulphanilamide belonged to the general commonwealth, not to any one company.

Colebrook continued cautiously to test Prontosil. In a further series of sixty-four women he showed a death rate of under 5 per cent. In another group of a hundred, in which he used both Prontosil and the straight sulphanilamide, eight died. In every group of women in which he used one of these new drugs, the death rate was substantially lower than the 20-odd per cent seen before they had become available.

Why was Colebrook so slow to be satisfied? Partly, it was because this thoughtful man found himself in agreement with the Scottish doctor John Cowan. Puerperal fever was more lethal than pneumonia. So in none of his examinations of the new drugs did Colebrook include a group of control women, of patients with puerperal fever to whom he deliberately denied the drug. It simply seemed to him to be too cruel.

That left him, however, with alternative explanations for the improvements he was seeing. What if the streptococcus was becoming spontaneously less hazardous, happening to evolve in a benign direction at the same time as these new compounds were being introduced? It sounded remarkably unlikely but there were reasons to take it seriously. Scarlet fever appeared to be doing exactly that, and it was a disease caused by the same streptococcus. Looking at the records of other hospitals, it was apparent to Colebrook that death rates from puerperal fever *were* declining, both before and during the introduction of these new sulfa drugs. And there was also reason to worry that the drugs themselves were dangerous. Colebrook found that a number of women treated with them suffered a change in the colour of their skin. It became dusky, dark and blue – a sign associated with potentially fatal changes in the blood's ability to carry oxygen and carbon dioxide.

Colebrook achieved two vital things. His series of 1936 papers in the *Lancet* meant that more admiring attention began to be paid to the sulfa drugs, and their popularity spread. His assertion of lingering uncertainty was also taken seriously. Colebrook managed to provoke not only useful enthusiasm but also fertile doubt. Further studies during the 1930s continued to look at the effects of sulfa drugs on puerperal fever. All of them were positive. Even though none used control groups (relying instead on the historical records from before the introduction of the sulfa drugs) they were persuasive.*

What became apparent to doctors, as a result of the introduction of sulfa drugs, was that the sort of proof a drug required depended on the magnitude of the benefit it offered. In puerperal fever and, from 1938 onwards, meningococcal meningitis, the diseases were so fatal and the drug so effective that certainty was relatively easy to come by. Comparing what happened at a hospital before and after a drug was introduced was likely to be reliable. For other infections, however, sulfa drugs were harder to figure out. Not only did most people with pneumonia recover anyway, for example, but rates of pneumonic infections also varied hugely from month to month and year to year. Subtler methods were needed to determine what impact sulfa drugs had on such comparatively mild diseases. In scarlet fever, doctors used concurrent controls, giving the sulfa to some people and not to others. The drug had no effect. That was a surprising finding. Reasoning logically, doctors assumed it was going to be useful – scarlet fever was caused, after all, by the same bug as puerperal fever. Despite that, there seemed to be no effect at all. Logic and reason were proving no match for experiment.

Before Domagk and Colebrook's work, one in every 500 births in Britain led to the mother's death. Knowing that the disease was sometimes spread by the hands of doctors and nurses had helped reduce rates, but not terrifically. Death rates had remained largely static over the previous eighty years. By 1940, after Prontosil, the death rate fell to one in 2,000.

* There was a paradox here. Colebrook felt that control groups were unethical for such a dangerous disease. He was unwilling to take the risks with women's lives that they entailed. The result was that acceptance of the drug's effects was slow. Far fewer women might actually have died had Colebrook used controls to begin with. By trying to avoid harm to a few, Colebrook inflicted it on many.

*

The French suggestion about the irrelevance of Prontosil rubrum's colouring to its activity turned out to be correct. Sulphanilamide was the portion of the compound with anti-bacterial activity. Fortunately for Farben, enough doctors ignored this fact to make the dye-based drug highly profitable. They seemed attached to Prontosil's name rather than its actions, choosing Prontosil rubrum over sulphanilamide in exactly the way that they had previously prescribed Antifebrin in place of acetanilide.*

In the meantime, Domagk himself got to use the drug. His six-year-old daughter Hildegarde was making Christmas decorations early in December 1935. Wanting help threading a needle, she carried it downstairs to look for her mother. She fell while carrying it carefully, as children are taught to do, with the sharp end pointing downwards and away from her. She landed badly enough that although the blunt eye of the needle was the part pressed against her palm, it was driven deep into her hand, sticking into the bone where the metal snapped in two.

After an X-ray, a surgeon removed the broken needle. The next day Hildegarde was feverish. An abscess developed where the metal had pricked her. Despite repeated surgical drainage of the pus, the infection grew worse. It spread from her hand into her arm. In a state of septic shock – her blood pressure desperately low as a result of the bacterial toxins – she became delirious. The surgeons talked about cutting her arm off in an attempt to save her life. Samples of her blood grew streptococcus. She was plainly dying.

Asking permission from the surgeon looking after her, Domagk fed his daughter Prontosil, putting the tablets in her mouth and watching while she swallowed them. Her recovery was quick and, by

* The same preference exists in the marketplace today. Ibuprofen tablets, for example, are available over the counter at chemists at very much cheaper prices than branded versions of the same thing, like Nurofen.

the standards of the day, wholly miraculous. By Christmas she was back at home, healthy.

Gerhard Domagk's smaller reward was the Nobel, in 1939. It came four years after Hitler forbade Germans from receiving these prizes. The 1935 Peace Prize had been awarded to Carl von Ossietzky, a pacifist critical of the Nazis. This had infuriated Hitler. In 1938 Ossietzky died in his concentration camp, his death doing nothing to lift the ban. When Domagk carefully acknowledged the award, thanking the committee but saying he was not sure if he could accept, it seemed far too polite a response in the eyes of the German authorities. Domagk was taken away by the Gestapo. After a period in jail, he was released. Travelling to Berlin to give a talk, he heard his name being called over the loudspeakers at the railway station in Potsdam. The Gestapo were waiting for him again, and told him there would be no talk. They offered him a letter declining the Nobel. He signed.

Domagk finally collected his prize in 1947. By then the money, according to the rules of the Nobel Foundation, was forfeit. Domagk accepted the prize anyway.

14   Penicillin and Streptomycin

To the extent that sulphonamides turned out to act independently of their staining power, their development was partly accidental. It was reminiscent of the sorts of accident that had led to cinchona replacing Peruvian balsam for treating malaria, or the Reverend Stone selecting willow bark for fevers on the basis that the tree grew in swamps. In the two older examples, though, a mistaken theory had led by good fortune to a happy outcome. Ehrlich and Domagk had done something different. Their study of dyes led them, correctly, to the idea that a compound might have selective toxicity for different organisms. Starting with dyestuffs was sensible, both because they had already been shown to enter bacteria and specific cell types, but also because their visual nature made them relatively easy to monitor. Actually, though, the development of antibiotics depended only on two things: that people could correctly conceive of them, and that a system could be put in place for screening large numbers of molecules in order to seek them out. Prontosil rubrum, by sheer chance, did not have to be red to work.

A huge group of scientists worked in Domagk's laboratory, testing one compound after another for its ability to save deliberately sickened and infected animals. That seems like a long way from the ideas of science that had begun to emerge in the seventeenth century. It was not. Francis Bacon, looking ahead, had seen that science was not for an elite only, that science 'is not a way over which only one man can pass at a time . . . but one in which the labours and industries of men (especially as regards the collecting of experience), may with the best effect be first distributed and then combined. For then only will men begin to know their strength.' That communal effort, more than any one person's inspiration, was behind the discovery of antibiotics.

During the First World War, Lieutenant (later Captain) Alexander Fleming spent time in France. Fleming worked to try to understand why war wounds went bad so often. The bandages soaked in antiseptic, so effective for the British during the Boer War, seemed to have little effect in Flanders. Wounds on the Western Front, Fleming found, were filthier. The mud and the high-velocity armaments drove dirt deep into damaged bodies, and oddly, as Fleming showed, washing out wounds with antiseptics did more harm than good. What seemed a reasonable approach was actually making things worse. The antiseptics killed lots of bacteria in wounds but they also killed the body's own cells. And the wounded depended on those for their ability to heal. Even the latest antiseptic technology cost lives if it was put into practice without being soundly tested first.

In the summer of 1928, while working in London, Fleming started experimenting with a mould. His actual interests at that stage were in lysozymes, a group of enzymes found in snot and other bodily fluids that were able to dissolve bacteria. The lysozymes had no effect on *Staphylococci*, a common bacterium in humans, but the mould did.

It was not a novel, surprising or even a particularly interesting finding. Mould's ability to kill bacteria had been described in 1876, by John Tyndall. He watched a piece of mutton rot, noting that the bacteria that grew on it were all killed by the mould. Like Fleming, Tyndall knew that he was observing the effects of a mould called *Penicillium*. 'In every case where the mould was thick and coherent,' Tyndall wrote, 'the Bacteria died, or became dormant.'

141

That made *Penicillium* no different in concept to carbolic acid, bleach or the other antiseptics. Fleming's official biographer noted the routine nature of what occurred, explaining that Fleming observed a mould that appeared to kill bacteria: 'probably the mould was producing acids which were harmful to the staphylococci – no unusual occurrence.' It was not an important event.

A far more astonishing demonstration of *Penicillium*'s properties had already come in 1897. A Frenchman named Ernest Duchesne submitted a doctoral thesis on the competition between micro-organisms, the battles they waged in order to live. '*Contribution à l'étude de la concurrence vitale chez les microorganismes – Antagonisme entre les moisissures et les microbes*' was a remarkable work. Duchesne claimed to have shown that injections of his *Penicillium* safely cured typhoid in animals. Unfortunately Duchesne's conclusions were rejected by the Pasteur Institute, his ideas had no impact, and it is not possible now to be certain about his methods. Whether his injections actually did work cannot be known. His understanding of what he was close to, however, is unmistakable. 'The question of vital competition was indeed studied up until now only for the higher animals and plants,' he wrote:

> It is not without interest to see whether, at the level of the infinitely small ones, this struggle for existence does not also exist, and whether it provides concepts useful for pathology or for therapeutics. The role of microbes in the genesis of disease is now well-known to us: we know that, not only do they generate disease, but they can also be the remedy for it, either by their attenuated culture or by products that they secrete.

Duchesne concluded that *Penicillium*, injected at the same time as a dose of typhoid, made the latter harmless. He thought that this was important. He died of tuberculosis in 1912, at the age of thirty-seven, without having convinced anyone or having continued his own work beyond his widely ignored doctorate.

Others had also noted the way in which penicillin killed bacteria. Like Fleming, they spared a thought for the possibility that this could be useful. 'Life hinders life,' Pasteur wrote in 1877. 'A liquid invaded by an organised ferment, or by an aerobe, makes it difficult for an inferior organism to multiply . . . These facts may, perhaps, justify the greatest hope from the therapeutic point of view.' The notion of simple organisms competing with others through chemical attacks was christened in 1899. Jean-Paul Vuillemin described how moulds fought with bacteria: 'Here there is nothing equivocal; one creature destroys the life of the other. The conception is so simple that no one has ever thought of giving it a name.' He called it antibiosis. A host of other nineteenth-century workers, including Lister, noted this ability of moulds to poison bacteria. In the same year that Pasteur wrote about his hopes, Lister even tried using *Penicillium* mould to treat infected wounds. He gave it up as hopeless.

Fleming attempted to purify the bacteria-killing substance that the mould produced. He was unsuccessful. Nevertheless he took steps that moved him closer to realising that 'the greatest hope' of mankind was sitting in the culture dishes on his laboratory bench. The extracts of mould juice that he made were not toxic either to white blood cells or to living mice. That made them exceptionally different from the antiseptics that people slapped onto operating theatre floors or soaked wound dressings in. It was not a difference, however, that greatly impinged on Fleming.

Fleming might have tested his 'penicillin' (a name he came up with early in 1929) on an infected animal, just as Domagk's laboratory took pains to do in the same year with their pigments. Animal activists at the time, however, argued forcefully that you could not learn about treating human diseases by trying remedies on rabbits or mice. From the middle of the nineteenth century, public opinion in

Britain in particular was appalled at the number of pointless vivisections carried out by doctors in the name of discovery. Astute observers pointed out that the vivisections almost never led to any new therapies, or to freshly effective treatments. Injecting his penicillin into deliberately infected laboratory animals was simply not something that occurred to Fleming as useful. Here, as well as in making the most of dyestuffs, the Germans led the way.

Knowing that his extracts were too full of impurities to be injected safely into humans, Fleming tried using his penicillin as a wound dressing. He put it on the infected stump of a woman's leg. It was no use. Fleming published a 1929 paper 'On the Antibacterial Action of Cultures of a Penicillium with Special Reference to Their Use in the Isolation of B. Influenzae'. Because penicillin killed most bacteria, he explained that it was superb at leaving the research clinician with culture plates free of everything except *B. influenzae*. That was a boon to those who wanted to explore the nature of this particular bug, but of no therapeutic use to anyone at all. Fleming moved on to other things, keeping cultures of penicillin growing in order to clean bacteria from his laboratory equipment, as his paper described. Various accounts have him occasionally using, and talking of, penicillin as the 1930s swept by and sulphonamides came onto the market. If he did talk to people about his belief that penicillin might be of great human value, and occasionally use his extracts of it to treat simple skin and eye infections, it only makes his overall inactivity more puzzling. Given the harms that doctors inflicted without realising, though, perhaps it should not be surprising to find them also being blind to benefits.

As a medical student in London in the 1920s, Cecil George Paine heard about penicillin from Fleming's lectures. When Paine started work in Sheffield he wrote and asked Fleming for some samples of the *Penicillium* mould. During 1930 and 1931, Paine tried it out. He gave extracts of the mould juice to three patients with skin infections, seeing no benefits. 'The attempts to use penicillin against these infections', said Paine, 'came to nothing.' He turned to using it on babies born with gonorrhoea. Although this was a sexually trans-mitted disease, an infant could pick up gonorrhoea in the process of being born. It affected the baby's eyes, filling them with infected pus. In one surviving set of medical notes, penicillin broth was applied to the eyes of a three-month-old named Peter. An inpatient since the age of three weeks, Peter was undergoing treatment with silver nitrate drops for his infected eyes.* On 25 November 1930 the notes say: 'Started c. Pinicillin' (*sic*). By 2 December, both eyes had cleaned up. The penicillin, remembered Paine, 'worked like a charm!'

Paine's mould was grown on meat broth, and like Fleming he was unable to manufacture any pure extracts of the broth's active ingredient. He simply used the broth in its entirety. Nevertheless, his experiments continued. A patient came in from one of the nearby mines, his eye pierced with a fragment of stone driven underneath his iris. The wound was infected, and Paine was able to swab the emerging pus and show which bacteria were living inside the man's eye. 'We took a culture from his cornea and grew up the organism that was absolutely dreaded in the eye – *Pneumococcus*,' said Paine. Operating on an infected wound was only done in order to cut out the infection entirely. Opening up the eye to remove the stone was simply likely to spread the infection. Removing the whole globe of the eye, before the infection spread back into the man's brain, seemed the best way forward. Instead, Paine and his colleagues took a different approach. 'We tried penicillin and it cleared up the infection like nobody's business, and they were able to deal with him and he made a good recovery.' With the infection cleared from his eye, the surgeons safely removed the stone. The man recovered and his vision returned to normal.

* Silver nitrate eye-drops have since been shown to be useless for this condition.

145

At the end of March 1931, Paine left to study puerperal fever with Leonard Colebrook in London, later returning to Sheffield to work at a women's hospital. He never again experimented with penicillin and did not publish accounts of his few trials of it.

Milton Wainwright and Harold Swan interviewed Paine towards the end of his life. They concluded that 'Paine had obviously seen a therapeutic potential in penicillin, although mainly in relation to its use as an antiseptic, but he was beaten by the unstable nature and variability of the crude extract'. It seems a fair summary. Paine's own verdict on himself was harsher, and quite different. Wainwright and Swan asked Paine where he saw himself fitting in to the story of penicillin's discovery.

'Nowhere', he replied:

a poor fool who didn't see the obvious when it was stuck in front of him. I suppose that there are many things that conspired to stop me doing it. I'm sorry, but there it is. It might have come on to the world a little earlier if I'd had any luck.

What Paine was suggesting was also, in its way, very fair. If you are going to acknowledge people who make discoveries, you also have to acknowledge those who came close but failed, those who 'didn't see the obvious when it was stuck in front of' them. Paine's sadness does not seem to have been for having missed out on fame and fortune. It was for the death and suffering that might have been avoided if he had achieved what others – including giants like Lister and Pasteur – also failed at.

Domagk's success with sulfonamides helped make penicillin achievable. Seeing his work, people turned to thinking about the production of other drugs with antibiotic properties. In Oxford, during the Second World War, a remarkable group of researchers took the *Penicillium* mould and reliably extracted pure concentrations of the molecule that gave it antibacterial activity. They were led by Howard Florey, an Australian Rhodes scholar who arrived at Magdalen College with burning intelligence, great ambition and a terror of the ways in which a man could fail in the world.

'I can see myself developing into a rather nasty product,' he wrote back to his sweetheart, herself a doctor.

> I'm that most damnably lonely I don't know what to do, sometimes. I'm not complaining against anyone or anything . . . but the fact is I haven't really got a friend as I conceive the term, and am quite incapable of having one.

Florey found people to support and encourage him, however, even if others shared the view that his greatest gifts were not social ones. 'Florey had a rather abrasive personality,' noted a colleague. 'He wouldn't call a spade a spade but he'd call it a bloody shovel.'

With Ernst Chain and Norman Heatley, Florey drove the development of penicillin as a drug. Much acclaim ended up going to Fleming, once the world began to realise the power of penicillin. Fleming was willing to give interviews, Florey was not. Fleming was well connected in London, and his supporters were quick to claim a greater share of the credit for him than he deserved. Newspaper journalists, more interested in writing quickly than writing truthfully, were happy to simplify and distort the story. Fleming himself did not go out of his way to attract extra credit, but made little effort to refuse it.

Out of the Oxford group, only Chain seemed to possess a genuine lust for fame, and a consequent grudge over history cheating him. Florey was angry at the misrepresentation, but his desire to put people right was calmer than Chain's. 'Nor should anyone suppose that we have performed any great intellectual feats here,' he wrote to

Britain's Medical Research Council, while asking them to make the drug's history clear. 'All we did was to do some decent experiments and have the luck to hit on a substance with astonishing properties.' Norman Heatley agreed: 'There wasn't anything original in it. It was a question of: here is a product; here is a method of making something. What is the something? How do you make it? . . . It was just a question of applying already-known techniques.'

The problem of credit could have been avoided, as Eric Lax pointed out in *The Mould in Dr Florey's Coat*, if the Oxford group had simply called their drug something different from 'penicillin'. Fleming originally used the name partly *because* of his own inability to figure out what substance within his mould juice was having an antibacterial effect. For him, 'penicillin' meant a poorly understood mix of fungal broth. The compound that Florey and his team isolated and mass-produced was something quite different, just as Aspirin was different from a piece of willow bark. Branding could – and should – have made all the difference.

The development of penicillin was a wartime adventure. Chief among the worries of the Oxford team was what might happen to their work in the event of a successful German invasion. For some time, that seemed far more likely than not. The title of Lax's book referred to the plan Florey and his colleagues developed during the bleakest days of the Second World War, when Britain's defeat looked close at hand. They intended to destroy their laboratories and burn their records, in order that the potential of penicillin should not fall into the hands of Hitler's Reich. As in the world's previous conflicts, disease as much as weaponry could decide the ultimate outcome of war. Florey, Chain, Heatley and others planned to rub *Penicillium* mould into their clothes, then try to escape. Their hope was that one of them, at least, might survive and reach a free country where they could continue their work.

The country they had in mind was America. Though they never needed to seek asylum there, American support for penicillin still proved vital. Florey's group was supported from an early stage – 1936 – by American money, filling gaps left by a lack of British funding.

William Osler's *Principles and Practice of Medicine*, first published in 1892 and the medical world's leading textbook for several decades after, had brought home to the medical community that their advances in understanding diseases were not matched by therapeutic breakthroughs. Osler's famed 'therapeutic nihilism', the scepticism about the value of therapy that he held in common with his friend Oliver Wendell Holmes, was provocative. (It was also far from complete, as shown by Osler's continued belief in the value of bleeding to treat pneumonia.) *Principles and Practice* played a key part in the influencing the aims of Rockefeller's rich philanthropic foundation. Founded in 1913 and endowed with $100 million by the following year, the Rockefeller Foundation showed an explicit interest in responding to Osler's proclamation that the world lacked effective medical drugs. One of the ways that interest manifested itself was in financial support for Florey's group in Oxford.

Penicillin, rather than the mould or its crudely gathered juice, was first used in Oxford's Radcliffe Infirmary in January 1941. Elva Akers, dying of cancer, was asked if she was willing to submit to an experimental dose of the stuff. There was no suggestion that it might do her any good – the point was that she was dying anyway. Was she willing to help? She was, and the drug did her no obvious harm.

Since it seemed safe, it was next given to an Oxfordshire policeman. The previous September, spending a quiet hour in his garden, he had scratched his cheek on a rose thorn. By February he was dying, his body riddled with infected abscesses, his left eye having been replaced by pus and then cut away entirely by surgeons. He responded beautifully to the penicillin, improving almost literally overnight. The drug was well on its way to saving his life when supplies, including those gathered by recrystallising it from his urine, ran out. He died.

Producing more in their university laboratory, the British team achieved properly successful human trials, curing other patients whose infections were clearly killing them. Despite their greatest attempts, though, they only managed to make enough of the drug for a handful of people. The *Penicillium* mould turned out such a small amount of the active drug that even their best methods of mass-production resulted in only tiny amounts of pure penicillin. British pharmaceutical companies, stretched by the war, were unwilling and unable to take much interest. So the Rockefeller Foundation flew Florey and Heatley to the USA. Florey stayed long enough to convince people, then returned to Oxford. Heatley, who knew most about actually growing and purifying penicillin, stayed longer.

He was there in March 1942, when penicillin was first used successfully in America. Anne Miller, thirty-three years old, was dying of a bacterial infection following a miscarriage – effectively a form of puerperal fever. Despite sulphonamides, the disease could still kill. Anne Miller was dying, however, in Yale, and that made all the difference. A fellow patient knew of penicillin, and at her doctor's request contacted the authorities that controlled the drug's wartime use. The pharmaceutical company Merck released a teaspoonful of the drug. At that stage, despite the efforts and investment of Merck and other companies, that teaspoonful was roughly half of the world's supply.

Norman Heatley, despite being the only person in America with clinical experience of penicillin, was not medically qualified. His background was pure science, and his morals and his Englishness made him feel that it was not his place to advise doctors. His private diaries, quoted in Lax's history of penicillin, give a flavour of the result. The Yale physician John Bumstead was amazed by Anne

Miller's marvellous response to penicillin. Wary of the drug, he wanted to reduce the dose as quickly as possible. Heatley, recalling the Oxford policeman whose disease fatally recurred when his penicillin ran out, disagreed, but could not quite bring himself to say so. Bumstead was acute enough to understand that Heatley was motivated by modesty, not ignorance. So, doggedly, he pursued the Englishman.

> Each day Bumstead asked Heatley, 'What would you recommend? Should we carry on with the penicillin?' And every time, Heatley answered, 'Look, I'm not medically qualified. It would be quite unethical for me to suggest anything.' So Bumstead would ask, 'Well, what do you think Dr Florey would say?' And Heatley would answer brightly, 'Oh, I think he would say carry on. You know, you can't stop it now.'

Anne Miller's therapy continued, the penicillin lasted, and she recovered completely. Later, as the power of penicillin became clear, the industrial production of it became part of the American war effort. By 1943 penicillin was America's second highest research priority. The only thing ahead of it was the Manhattan Project.

By D-Day the United States was manufacturing enough penicillin each month to treat 40,000 people – enough to have, as everyone had hoped, a significant effect on wartime fatalities.

Penicillin's success saved lives and encouraged research. It also cemented in the minds of doctors the belief that you could figure out what a drug did simply by giving it and seeing what happened. It was, after all, a genuine miracle drug, a wonder. Its good effects were of such a magnitude there was no mistaking them and, by chance, it was remarkably safe. Doctors too easily concluded that science was providing them with such new and marvellous cures, that there was no need to engage in any complicated weighing-up of risks, no requirement to think carefully about balancing harms and benefits: no need to be scientists themselves.

Merck, one amongst many drug companies who were impressed by this experience of penicillin, immediately started looking for similar drugs. They were far from the only ones to do so, but they were certainly one of the most successful. Merck had continued to be a family firm from its inception in 1668 through to George Merck setting up an American branch in 1891. His son, George W. Merck, graduated from Harvard in 1915 – a time when his plan for returning to Germany to engage in research was particularly impractical. Instead he started straight away, working for the family company. In 1917, as a result of the war, it became a legally separate entity from its German parent. A Merck, however, was still in charge.

During the Second World War, George W. Merck showed his patriotism and his power. He did everything he could to help America win the war through pharmaceuticals. That meant sulfonamides, penicillin and, at Camp Detrick in Maryland, germ warfare.

One of Merck's efforts at discovering new antibiotics lay in the company's funding of Selman Waksman. A Russian émigré, Waksman's academic interest at Rutgers University was in soil microbiology. Inspired by penicillin, Waksman focused on trying to extract antibacterial compounds from the microscopic life that soil was packed with. In human terms, they were part of the carbon cycle, breaking down detritus and making the earth fertile. In their own terms, they were engaged in the same sort of battle for survival as every other creature – and germ warfare was one of the ways in which they fought too.

In 1942, Waksman took on a doctoral student named Albert Schatz. Schatz's studies were interrupted by the war, but not for long. Within a year he was discharged from the army, a bad back making him ineligible for active duty. He returned to Waksman. The arrangements that the two men made, like other aspects of their relationship, are now subject to disagreement. Some accounts say that Schatz spent his army months watching men die from tuberculosis, arriving back at Rutgers and insisting on being allowed to look for a cure. Others describe him agreeing to work on antibiotic research only because Waksman made it a condition of his getting paid.

The ill feeling between the two men was based on what happened in October of 1943. After studying Waksman's soil samples for only a few months, Schatz discovered a new antibiotic. Others had been found before in soil, but they had proven too toxic for human use. This one – streptomycin – was different. Waksman, having set up the programme of soil testing but taken no part in Schatz's day-to-day laboratory work, arranged for the new compound to be tested at the Mayo Clinic. It was given to four tuberculous guinea pigs. None were cured, but their disease was significantly subdued and the drug seemed to do them no harm. It was an impressive result, suggesting real potential. Waksman pressured Merck into calling a board meeting. He wanted the company to back further research into the drug, an expensive business. The board members were reluctant to agree. Then George W. arrived, late, to the meeting. He supported Waksman's idea wholeheartedly.*

In the way it affected bugs, streptomycin turned out to be very different from penicillin. It did not kill them, only stopped them from reproducing. That seemed to be enough, though, to allow the body's immune system to get the upper hand. Waksman travelled to the Mayo Clinic to explain the story so far at first hand. 'In September 1943,' he told his audience, 'my assistants and I succeeded in isolating in our laboratory an organism that produced an antibiotic.' Thereafter he was even less charitable, often failing to mention

---

* He later donated all of Merck's international patent rights in streptomycin to Rutgers.

Schatz at all. The rancour between the two men grew. Waksman continued to receive the credit and the benefits of the discovery, going on to become rich from the patent and ennobled by a Nobel prize. Schatz, in contrast, finished his life sharpening knives in Philadelphia, feeling bitter and cheated. 'Thou shalt not take the credit for thy junior collaborators' work,' was the verdict of the Nobel laureate Max Perutz, who wrote about the controversy. Waksman collected the soil organisms and set up the machinery to study them, but Schatz was lucky enough to stumble across exactly the right one. The notion that an element of luck made someone ineligible for credit was ludicrous, at least to Perutz, who knew from experience how vital good fortune was for scientific discovery.

The corporate nature of scientific research, in which credit often deserved to be shared, was sometimes difficult for scientists to acknowledge. Waksman seems to have imagined that he and Schatz belonged to a system where all credit was due to the leader who sat at the top (almost literally: while Schatz was in the basement doing his experiments, Waksman was sitting above in his office). Of more concern to patients than the priority for discovery, however, were emerging doubts over exactly what it was that the new drug offered.

Measurements of its concentration in blood showed little correlation between how much a patient was given and the quantity that flowed around their body. That was worrying, since streptomycin was clearly dangerous, damaging nerves and kidneys and destroying people's hearing. Yet the experiments on guinea pigs continued to be promising, and streptomycin very much seemed like the sort of thing that ought to work. On the back of the success of sulphonamides and penicillin, the blind conviction was that anti-biotics were good things. Without further trials, America adopted the drug enthusiastically.

Even at the time, people should have known better. The unquestioning use of streptomycin was not rational: it was an example of the optimism with which doctors and patients had been dosing themselves for thousands of years. By the middle of the twentieth century, it should have been clear that there were more sensible ways of behaving. Even within the treatment of tuberculosis, there were recent lessons.

Another new drug of the time was Sanocrysin, a gold-based compound. Developed in Denmark, it became popular in America from the middle of the 1920s. Gold was known to be thoroughly toxic, but then tuberculosis was dangerous and the benefits of the drug were felt to outweigh its harms. In 1925 the *American Journal of Public Health* managed to reserve a little judgement over the new therapy, but approved all the same of doctors using it on the basis of good reports from Europe. 'It can be said of this alleged cure that it is being given to the public in a thoroughly professional manner,' it decided. The *Canadian Medical Journal*, in 1927, held a similar opinion, suggesting that although the proper dose of the drug was not yet established, it was clearly beneficial.

Other doctors managed to disagree, but since they focused on the patients who did badly, while the drug's supporters dwelt on those who did well, neither side could persuade the other. Not until 1931 was the drug tested with any degree of reliability. In Detroit, an unusually thoughtful group of doctors took twenty-four tuberculous patients and tried to split them into two equally matched groups. 'Obviously, the matching could not be precise, but it was as close as possible, each patient having previously been studied independently by two of us.' With a flip of a coin, one group was allocated to Sanocrysin and the other to nothing. The doctors running the trial took care to hide the allocation from the patients and the other staff. They gave everyone either Sanocrysin, or similar looking injections that were actually nothing but sterile water.

The Detroit study showed that the patients given the water were more likely to survive than those given the Sanocrysin. The wonderfully promising drug, in other words, did more harm than good.

The same issue of the *American Review of Tuberculosis* that published the Detroit report also contained another study, this time from a tuberculosis sanatorium in Kentucky. There a doctor told of giving Sanocrysin to a group of forty-six people. He used no control group, and his conclusion was that the drug was 'outstanding'. The presence of the two reports in the same publication provided the best possible affirmation that careful trials and control groups, particularly when it came to dangerous drugs and unpredictable diseases like tuberculosis, were absolutely essential.

This should have meant a great deal to the early adopters of streptomycin. Instead it was ignored. The new antibiotic had to wait for further advances in the way doctors weighed up the effects of their drugs, advances that were to come mainly from Britain.

15 'Sickness in Salonica: my first, worst and most successful clinical trial'

Thoughtful approaches to figuring out what worked emerged slowly, gradually, and without clear direction. Innovations were ignored, insights passed by, developments left to lead nowhere. Improvements in testing showed no tendency to come together as a trend, a movement, something infectious and impulsively self-propagating. Even tests that sound startlingly modern were often less advanced than they seemed. The work of James Lind is a good example.

Lind is often held up as the man who invented the reliable clinical trial. Born in 1716 in Edinburgh, Lind became a doctor for the Royal Navy, then greatly troubled by scurvy. The causes of the disease were a mystery, but its effects were well known. Gums bled, teeth and hair fell out, old wounds reopened and ulcers appeared where no wound had ever been. Delusions and hallucinations, bleeding and joint problems, blindness and death: scurvy was a miserable condition.

In 1740, Commodore Anson set out to circumnavigate the globe in order to attack the Spanish in South America. Out of a total crew of 1,900 in six vessels, only 400 survived. The majority were killed by scurvy. The account of the journey, published to literary acclaim in 1748, drew public attention. According to Lind's survey, the disease killed more Royal Navy sailors than died in armed conflict. He saw scurvy at first hand, sailing in afflicted ships from the 1730s. Lind wrote that his interest in the disease was stimulated by the account of Anson's voyage. That was possibly a politically astute comment, since Anson rose to become First Lord of the Admiralty. The timing suggests it was not wholly true. The incident for which Lind is praised took place in 1747, the year before publication of the book that was supposed to have inspired it.

Lind was on board the *Salisbury*, part of the Channel Fleet. With a crew of 350, the ship sailed for ten weeks. Before the voyage was over, eighty sailors were suffering from scurvy. On 20 May 1747, Lind took twelve of these men and divided them into pairs. 'Their cases were as similar as I could have them. They all in general had putrid gums, the spots and lassitude, with weakness of their knees. They lay together in one place, being a proper apartment for the sick in the fore-hold.' Lind gave each pair a different treatment: vinegar, cider, sulphuric acid, sea water, a paste made from herbs and Peruvian balsam bark, or citrus fruit. The two who received the fruit made rapid and remarkable recoveries, while the others did not. Read about Lind and you are likely to be told that this was not only the origin of proper trials, but also the experiment that saved sailors from scurvy by demonstrating the powers of fresh citrus.

Neither is true. Lind was behaving in what sounds a modern way, but had no real understanding of what he was doing. That made a difference. He failed so completely to make sense of his own experiment that even he was left unconvinced of the exceptional benefits of lemons and limes. Unsurprisingly, that meant he convinced no one else of them. People carried on dying of scurvy and doctors, including Lind, continued blindly guessing at treatments without realising they had the methods at hand to actually test them.

Nevertheless, something in Lind's behaviour was important. Not in the manner of a discovery, flashing out upon the world and changing it for ever. More after the style of a thought floating in the air, past a man who caught at and almost kept hold of it. Nearly two centuries later, in the years before the Second World War, ideas about trials were seeping into people's consciousness with new power. Lind was being increasingly held up as an example of something to aspire to, and even if that was based on a misunderstanding it said something important about what doctors were now learning to value. One of that new breed of doctors was a man named Archie Cochrane.

Archibald Leman Cochrane was born in 1909, growing up in Galashiels, in southern Scotland. His family were wealthy, he was intelligent, confident and from an early age showed both a love for sport and a dislike of unthinking authority. Sport dominated his early life, until he ripped the muscles of his right leg apart playing rugby at Cambridge. Temporarily crippled, he discovered a deep enjoyment of reading and thinking. It persisted once his leg healed.

An inability to ejaculate, as well genuine interest in the ideas of Freud, took him across Europe in pursuit of a psychoanalytic cure. Then he was off to the Spanish Civil War, refusing to sign up as a communist but believing that the Spanish republic was worth fighting for, and that fascists were worth fighting against.* Despite not having finished his medical studies, in 1936 Cochrane was nevertheless put in charge of the casualty clearing station at a small military hospital in Spain. There were more people there who needed medical help than there was help to give. That gave Cochrane a taste for rationing, for thinking about how to allocate scarce medical resources in the most efficient way possible. He noticed that one of the surgeons dealt with certain types of patients exceedingly slowly.

---

* 'I had one interesting meeting in a bar in Barcelona with a tall Englishman with big feet,' he remembered, but found George Orwell a difficult man to like. 'I later enjoyed his books more than I had that conversation.' Hemingway, whom he met around the same time, struck him as 'an alcoholic bore'.

'A nurse told me, as he did later, that he was not a very experienced abdominal surgeon. I then decided to give priority on his lists to orthopaedic cases and accept that some abdominal cases would consequently die. I think I was right.'

This was a fruitful start, as well as a mark of Cochrane's quality. He denied medical care to some people so that as many as possible would live. In his 1989 memoir, he told of the casualties arriving during one particular battle:

> The first case was lying on his right side with his face partially hidden. His left thorax was completely shattered. I could see a heart faintly beating. I signalled to the nurse, by dropping my thumb, that the case was hopeless (language was dangerous). I moved left to see the next case and, by chance, glanced back. To my horror I recognised the face of Julian Bell.

Too disturbed by the sight of his dying friend to trust his own judgement, Cochrane quickly got a second opinion. His colleague reassured him that his impulse was correct. The injuries were too severe. Acting humanely, when there was too little help to go around, meant abandoning people that could not be quickly helped with real hope of saving them. Julian was in Spain working as a volunteer ambulance driver for the republican forces. He died shortly afterwards from the effects of the bomb that had destroyed his chest.

Returning to England to finish his medical training, Cochrane was frightened that his year's absence, his new appearance and his left-wing sympathies would make the hospital reject him. Sunburnt and with 'a striking red Van Dyck beard', he nervously tested his reception, deliberately joining the ward round of University College Hospital's most right-wing physician. 'Ah, there you are, Cochrane,' was his greeting. 'How nice to see you. Had an interesting weekend?'

Noting the political convulsions in Germany, Cochrane loathed the prospect of Europe's descent into conflict but saw no way out. 'I had always considered that fascism had to be fought and that war was therefore inevitable. But I hated the idea of being involved in war again, knowing what it was like.' For Archie, when it came to both medicine and in politics, the fact that reality was harsh was no excuse for failing to face up to it.

After qualifying as a doctor, Cochrane helped University College Hospital prepare for casualties, and then he enrolled in the army. He was sent first to a field ambulance unit in Dorset and then, after a course at the London School of Hygiene and Tropical Medicine, was posted to Egypt. He sailed from Glasgow, finding companionship on the way with another doctor, Richard Doll. The two passed the voyage talking, organising concerts and studying Arabic. (Doll remembered their differences in approach. They studied, 'Archie from a large tome that began with the Arabic script and me from the Berlitz paperback *Teach Yourself Arabic in Three Months*.') After a period in Egypt, horrified at the conditions of the country's poor, Cochrane's language skills led him in a new direction. A commando battalion containing refugees from Spain needed a doctor; was he willing? He was. The physical demands of his new role as a commando were difficult, at least to begin with. 'I remember a particularly arduous long desert march,' Cochrane recalled, 'with limited water supplies. Colonel Young, for whom I developed a great respect, advised me to march just behind him and not to worry if I hallucinated.'

The battalion sailed to Crete, with the author Evelyn Waugh serving as intelligence officer. Cochrane was briefed by a senior officer on the mission: 'He told me, in a rather apologetic way, that casualties were going to be high and that as it was likely that I would be killed he was taking the unusual step of sending a second medical officer with the battalion.'

Cochrane survived, but the Allied invasion of Crete went

disastrously wrong. At the end of May the remaining Allied troops surrendered. Life as a prisoner of war started off haphazardly for Cochrane. As a doctor who spoke German fluently, he was thrust into responsibility. He struggled with hostile prisoners speaking a babble of languages, with conditions that were often appalling, and with sadism and murderousness from the German guards. Battered by indignity, exhaustion, hunger and loneliness, he fortified himself by holding ever more tightly to those things that he felt mattered most: his efforts to write poetry and to provide the best medical care he could.

Interned at Salonica, Cochrane watched as bodies and morals collapsed under the stress of starvation and imprisonment. Six hundred calories a day were too little. The toilets within the barrack houses were too poor and too few, and at night the prisoners were forbidden from using the extra ones immediately outside their huts. As July became August the Germans began shooting some of their prisoners, randomly and without reason. 'Then came a day I shall never forget,' said Cochrane. A New Zealand orderly was shot while working in the camp hospital. Then a Yugoslav orderly, then another New Zealander. One of the men died of his wounds. Cochrane, in a fury, demanded an audience with the camp *Kommandant*. He was refused. That night, hearing prisoners using the outside toilets, a guard threw in a hand grenade. It exploded in the middle of men trying to relieve themselves. The next morning the *Kommandant* publicly congratulated the guard.

That afternoon, Cochrane got his meeting:

I had recovered from my wild rage and decided to try another line. I said in fluent German – and in German I have a rather upper-class accent – how much I had admired German culture in the past. I mentioned the usual names – Goethe, Heine, Beethoven, and Mozart – and how much had been contributed to medicine through Robert Koch and, more recently, the discovery of the sulphonamides. How shocked I was therefore to find Germans, in breach of the Geneva Convention, trying to starve prisoners of war to death, murdering medical orderlies, and attempting to shoot doctors and dentists.

Shaming people into behaving more like human beings seemed to work. After Cochrane's outburst, the prisoners were treated better. Shootings stopped. Illnesses began to become the major problem. Cochrane was supplied with aspirin and a little quinine, but nothing else. Epidemics of diphtheria, typhoid and hepatitis began. 'I told those with typhoid to lie still on their own faeces and I would see they were well hydrated and given as much glucose as I could get out of the Germans.' Hepatitis actually became popular: while you were sick with it, you lost your appetite. That was a torment which hungry men were glad to be rid of.

As the summer passed, Cochrane noticed another condition appearing. Men's legs and ankles began to swell. It looked to be the result of famine, the same sort of process that bloats the bellies of babies dying of starvation. Cochrane begged to be allowed extra help – some blood tests and some senior medical advice – but the Germans refused him. 'Doctors are superfluous,' they told him.

The numbers of men affected by the swelling seemed to be increasing rapidly. Cochrane went to the camp's cooks and got figures for the number of men incarcerated, then used them to calculate day-to-day changes in rates of the disease. The numbers frightened him, and made him feel that some sort of action was essential. Persuading the Germans was more difficult.

In England, Cochrane had been taught the traditional story that James Lind had invented the clinical trial and saved the British Navy from scurvy. Inspired by that example, Cochrane took twenty of the prisoners, all with swelling rising up to their thighs. He divided them into two groups, installing each into a separate ward room of his camp hospital. To one he gave extra yeast supplements, bought on the black market with his own money. The others got vitamin C tablets.

> I expected, and feared, failure. I noted the numbers each morning. There was no difference between rooms for the first two days; on the third day there was a slight difference; and on the fourth it was definite.

The men taking yeast grew markedly better, a result that was remarkable for two reasons. First for the influence that Cochrane's findings gave him: his numbers appeared to have a persuasive power that his unaided complaints previously lacked. 'I suddenly realised that I had truly shaken the Germans.' Part of his success seemed to be down to the ghost of James Lind. The German doctors, too, came from universities where he was held up as a bright example.

The sheer passion of the odd-looking British doctor also had an effect. 'My face was emaciated and deeply jaundiced, but it was surrounded by a mass of red hair and an impressive red beard.' Cochrane's legs were swollen also, his own disease easily apparent. The Germans listened to him courteously and promised to help.

Despite his apparent success, Cochrane was worn out by worry and illness. He was convinced that his trial was wrong, that the cause of the swelling was not a shortage of yeast but just an overall famine of food. Ten people in each group were simply so few that an apparent difference had emerged by chance. Nothing real, just the effect of one group of ten happening to feel better than another. 'I returned to my room and wept. The outlook seemed helpless.'

The next day, though, was brighter. Not only did the Germans supply the yeast that had seemed to help, they also everyone's daily calories by a third. Health in the camp improved, and with it the morale of all the prisoners.

As regards the trial, I have always felt rather emotional about it and ashamed of it. I was testing the wrong hypothesis, the numbers were too small, and they were not randomised. The outcome measure was pitiful and the trial did not go on long enough. On the other hand, it could be described as my first, worst, and most successful trial.

Cochrane learnt that a bad trial can easily give a false result. He did not believe that it was lack of yeast that caused the illness, only lack of calories. He also took to heart the lesson that any trial at all, even a mistaken one, was the sort of thing that doctors were now being swayed by. They might not be able to distinguish good methods from bad, but they knew that methods mattered. That was a step forwards.

As the war went on, Cochrane was transferred from Greece into Germany, ending up at a camp at Elsterhorst. It was where the majority of tuberculous Allied prisoners were sent, and the treatment options available to the British doctors were reasonably broad. That is, they were largely the same as those available in the hospitals of the day. Tuberculosis could affect any part of the body; it took up most medical time when it affected the lungs. Since Koch's work the causative organism could be spotted in a patient's spit, but that did not solve the question of how to deal with it. The only available antibiotics, the sulphonamides, were of no use. At the camp, as in London, the doctors could prescribe bed-rest, a common treatment for tuberculosis. They could also deliberately deflate men's lungs. The idea was that the lungs could then rest, recovering from their infection. The British doctors were free to decide when such procedures should be undertaken. It was a freedom that troubled Cochrane. He became acutely aware that such decisions were never made on the basis of anything other than an individual doctor's personal opinions.

Even outside prison camps, tuberculosis was the developed world's biggest infectious killer of young men. And despite their relatively good medical care, a lot of the tuberculous prisoners died. The Germans had a policy, which Cochrane applauded, that the doctor caring for a patient was always in charge of organising the funeral. 'It was a good idea in that it brought home to physicians their case fatality rate.' Cochrane could see its benefit in terms of improving the accuracy of a doctor's experience; doctors too easily remembered their successes and forget about their failures. He also saw the human gain, the need to learn languages and religious customs, to grapple with the emotions as well as the therapeutics of looking after the very sick.

Part of the problem, he realised, was that the pressure to do something for the dying – anything at all – outweighed the need to take care that your actions did not make things worse. Cochrane began by trying to avoid deflating his patients' lungs, convinced that it could do more harm than good. Yet it was difficult: whenever he did intervene, his patients were glad of it. They longed to see their doctor *doing* something. Despite his awareness of doubt, despite the knowledge that he might well be making these patients worse, Cochrane found that deflating their lungs made him feel better too. The pressure to act, even for the worst, was overwhelming.

There were also times when what was required from a doctor was an entirely intuitive therapeutic intervention. Trials were not the only way of discovering what worked. At the end of a long day in Elsterhorst, the Germans handed over to Cochrane a young Soviet prisoner, screaming in pain and dying. Examining him, Cochrane found that tuberculosis had eaten up the man's lungs, and that the outer covering of one of them, the pleura, was inflamed. It rubbed agonisingly against the inside of the man's ribs each time he took a breath.

Unwilling to let the man's cries wake the ward, Cochrane

brought him into his own room and treated him there. Aspirin had no effect; there was no morphine available. The man's screams were awful. Cochrane knew a little Russian, but not enough, and there was no one who could translate. At last, unable to bear the man's howls any longer, Cochrane sat down on the bed and held him. The screams faded away. A little while later, apparently peacefully, the man died. The inflamed coverings of his lungs were not what had been most painful to the dying man: that had been loneliness and terror. 'It was a wonderful education about the care of the dying,' wrote Cochrane. 'I was ashamed of my [initial] misdiagnosis and kept the story secret.'

In January 1945 the Germans attempted to move some of the desperately sick tuberculous patients, loading them carelessly onto the open back of a truck while the snow came down. 'I had looked after these patients for a long time and had done my best. I loved them dearly. I thought this murder. I lost my temper and jumped on the wagon and made a loud speech to the Germans.' Their behaviour, he told them, was shameful: '*Das ist doch ein Skandal im Lande von Robert Koch*': 'This is a scandal in the land of Robert Koch.' The truck was replaced with an ambulance but Cochrane was dismissed from his post in the camp and replaced with another doctor.

By the end, Cochrane felt he had done as well as he was able. He was troubled, though, by the thought that he had shortened some of his patients' lives, not knowing the actual impacts of the medical choices he was making. The day-to-day demands of clinical work, he discovered, were also not enough for him. 'I had found it emotionally satisfying and distressing at the same time. I knew my patients so well that I was miserable when they died. I also found 'caring' intellectually unsatisfactory.' Had he been less of a man, had he been able to convince himself of his own power always to determine what was best, like when to deflate a lung, he would not have been left so unsatisfied. Cochrane clung successfully and painfully to an awareness of his own ignorance. It was something that only a minority of doctors before him seemed to have managed. It was something that came partly by virtue of his character, partly because the world in which he developed was beginning to change. Within the medical sciences, humility was spreading.

On 25 April 1945, some German civilians brought in a young girl with a badly damaged arm. In the filth and darkness of a cellar, Cochrane cut it off. When he emerged, he found that the guards were all gone. He was free.

Soon the Soviets arrived. Finding him dressing the German girl's stump of an arm, a Russian soldier informed Cochrane that he was to be shot for aiding the enemy. The threat was sincere, and the soldier meant to carry out his sentence immediately, but he allowed himself to be distracted by Cochrane's questions about his medals. Vanity got the upper hand. The American soldiers, when they arrived, seemed to Cochrane almost as bad. They were less violent, but they stole his belongings and showed a ready interest in rape. Being liberated was not such a pleasant experience.

When he got home, Cochrane found that the British army was not quite done with him. For some months after the war finished he worked in a military hospital in the small cathedral city of St Albans, running the tuberculosis ward. Then, funded by the same Rockefeller Foundation that enabled Florey's production of penicillin, Cochrane turned his back on clinical work and chose research instead. Prior to a period of training in Philadelphia, the Rockefeller Foundation sent him on a preparatory course at the London School of Hygiene and Tropical Medicine. There, from 1946 to 1947, Cochrane studied medical statistics under Austin Bradford Hill. The two men were to be instrumental in bringing to medicine an entirely novel degree of methodological rigour – changing the way doctors viewed the nature of evidence and having a more profound effect on human health than any newly discovered drug. One of the diseases on which their ideas most quickly had an effect was tuberculosis.

16   Captain of the Men of Death

By 1947, tuberculosis in Britain was only an eighth as common as it had been at the start of the century. It was not because treatments had improved, or the climate grown healthier. Better food and housing, as well as sanitation and hygiene, made people more resistant to *Mycobacterium tuberculosis*. Sulfonamides and penicillin, although they had no effect on the germ itself, helped by treating the added bacterial infections that TB sufferers were vulnerable to. In 1935, around 70,000 people died of tuberculosis in England and Wales. By 1947 it was only 55,000.

For centuries, ideas about testing had popped up here and there, only to have no apparent impact and to disappear for the span of an age. That, finally, was changing. The idea of using controls, and sample sizes big enough to overcome the flukes of chance, were taking root in the medical mind. By the time physicists were building nuclear weapons, doctors were conscious that reliable evidence only came from comparing groups that were significantly bigger than one person who took a drug and one who did not.

From Francis Galton onwards, progress formed a palpable chain of events. Not only did the methods for figuring medicines out improve rapidly, they did so in a sort of order. Francis Galton was idolised, and his work continued, by Karl Pearson. They met around the start of the twentieth century, when Pearson was forty and Galton eighty. It would be Galton, Pearson proclaimed, whom history would recognise as the greatest grandson of the eighteenth-century poet-physician Erasmus Darwin. The other competitor, Charles Darwin, was comparatively second-rate. The theory of evolution, to Pearson's mind, was infinitely less useful to humanity than a grasp of statistical method.

Pearson's work was broad, but the thrust of it was epistemological. How could people order their experience of the world in order to better understand it? How could they use numbers to help them think about the nature of things, explore the relationships between events, distinguish coincidence from causation? Pearson felt people were on the verge of new ways of understanding and dealing with the world. His radicalism was widespread. Beyond statistics and the theories of knowledge that went with it, he was passionately attached to other causes. Revolutionary socialism was one, and he combined it freely with a totalitarian view of eugenics and of racial differences, as well as a belief in the value of warfare for keeping the superior races pure.

Unsurprisingly, it was Pearson's brilliance that attracted people to him, not his human warmth. The young Einstein read him and recommended him to others. Pearson's impact was to turn statistics from an interest of gentleman amateurs into an academic discipline at the centre of scientific method. The chairs he held – Applied Mathematics and Mechanics at University College London, Geometry at the Royal Society's home of Gresham College – were ones whose names did not quite suit him. That was because statistics was not the sort of thing academia had ever taken seriously. In Pearson's wake, that changed.

An important ally was Major Greenwood, whose curious first name was not actually a title. Greenwood qualified as a doctor in 1904 at the age of twenty-four and, like Archie Cochrane, left clinical work behind as soon as he possibly could. He went to work instead with a physiologist in London, Leonard Hill. Hill's wife disapproved. 'I do hope', she declared to her husband, 'you are not going to appoint that cynical little man to your staff.' 'The boy has brains,' replied Leonard Hill. 'He'll never be any use as a doctor, and I must give him a chance in science.' Greenwood was soon writing articles for *Biometrika*, Karl Pearson's statistical journal, and went on to study with Pearson himself. The two men were comparable in their love of numbers, and perhaps also in the reasons why they found the world of mathematics attractive. 'Some have thought that he selected statistics as his life's work because that branch of medicine was most remote from the emotional,' explained a close friend of Greenwood's. 'Perhaps they were right.'

In 1928, now forty-eight, Greenwood was appointed to the first professorship in Epidemiology and Vital Statistics at the London School of Hygiene and Tropical Medicine. Like his election to the Royal Society, his professorial chair acknowledged the influence that statisticians were beginning to exert. Greenwood, declared his Royal Society nomination, 'has done much to encourage and develop the use of modern statistical methods by medical laboratory investigators, and, as Chairman of the Medical Research Council's Statistical Committee, to secure the adequate planning and execution of field investigations'.

Medical tests were becoming team efforts, just as pharmacology had been for almost a century. That meant there was a pressure for people to think about how they were organised, and an opportunity for those at the centre to control how the humble workers in the field collected and ordered their experiences and experiments. 'In the future,' read one of Greenwood's obituaries, 'it may well indeed seem that one of his greatest contributions, if not the greatest, lay merely in his outlook, in his statistical approach to medicine, then a new approach and one long regarded with suspicion. And he fought this fight continuously and honestly – for *logic*, for *accuracy*, for "*little sums*".' The obituary also noted that Greenwood's feeling for numbers was mixed with a clumsiness with people.

> To some he may have seemed distant and unapproachable, to some cynical and censorious. He was indeed not a person whom it was easy to get to know well . . . He was certainly censorious of pomposity and pretentiousness, and could be a devastating critic of the illogical and the stupid. In the medical journals his letters, epigrammatic and satirical, were widely read with enjoyment or pain – according to one's position.

The obituary writer was Austin Bradford Hill, the son of the physiologist Leonard. Born in 1897, at the close of the nineteenth century, Austin Bradford Hill grew up with the advantage of a father who was educated, thoughtful and attentive. Leonard Hill's publications included innovative physiological works, the auto-biographical *Philosophy of a Biologist* and, more usefully for Austin's childhood, *The Monkey Moo Book* and other collections of fairytales. The family home was a good place for a growing boy to learn that a feeling for numbers could fit perfectly well with human warmth.

When the First World War began Hill joined up as a pilot. The Royal Naval Air Service was officially formed in 1914, although the navy (offended at the army's control of the Royal Flying Corps, founded in 1912) had been operating it without permission for some time. Posted to Gallipoli in 1917, two years after the catastrophic British and Commonwealth battle to secure it, Hill travelled overland through France and Italy. By the time he reached the Aegean an attack of tuberculosis, possibly acquired en route, was so bad that he was sent straight home.

His tuberculosis was pulmonary, of the lungs, and that made it unpredictable. For a time it seemed likely to kill him. After two years in hospital, however, he emerged, debilitated but alive. Too weak to follow his father and obtain a medical degree, Hill spent a further two years convalescing before he became strong enough to look for work. At that point Major Greenwood stepped in, returning the support that Leonard Hill had once given him, and offered Austin a start in medical statistics. Working for the Medical Research Council, Hill studied statistics under Karl Pearson. Then, when Greenwood was made Professor of Epidemiology and Vital Statistics, he appointed Austin as Reader.

One of Hill's duties was teaching statistics to medics. It gave him an appreciation of just how difficult it was for doctors to tolerate the subject, let alone understand it. During the 1930s, he drew his lectures together into a series of articles, publishing them in the *Lancet*. Later they were collected and released as a book: *Principles of Medical Statistics*.

'Is the application of the numerical method to the subject-matter of medicine a trivial and time-wasting ingenuity as some hold, or is it an important stage in the development of our art, as others proclaim it?' the *Lancet* asked in 1921. Opinion in the medical profession was inclined to hope that it was the former. There was something much more comfortable about the days in which a doctor's sage opinions were considered sufficient, and the nuisance of numbers could be largely avoided. Hill's book noted this reluctance and did a fair job of patiently sympathising with it. At the same time it pointed out that doctors could not conscionably give in to it. Their tendency was to regard statistics as 'obscure and even repellent'. The obscurity had to be wiped away through hard work and study, while the repellent nature of statistics was something they had either to overcome or learn to put up with.

Statistics was now installing itself at the centre of medical research. That did not mean that the clinical community, mainly made up of doctors who finished their training before statistics bit into the curriculum, were already converted. Although medical papers were increasingly smattered with numbers, few of the researchers yet understood them. Controls and case series, percentages and other numerical measures were used as a form of dressing. Just as doctors once packed their writing with references to Galen and Hippocrates, now they did so with mathematical jargon. These meaningless mockeries of statistics added to the distrust doctors felt: many of the numbers filling medical journals and textbooks were patently nonsense.

Against these feelings, Hill argued that practical experience and wisdom were not enough to make sense of the way diseases behaved and treatments acted. 'Are simple methods of the interpretation of figures only a synonym for common sense or do they involve an art or knowledge which can be imparted?' he asked. 'Familiarity with medical statistics', he tempted doctors to believe, 'leads inevitably to the conclusion that common sense is *not* enough.' Hill was sensitive to frightening off any incipient interest. He was almost apologetic in his book, pointing out that what he had to say was so obvious it was barely worth saying – except, he added in the politest possible way, for the fact that doctors seemed unable to notice it for themselves.

Statistics, explained Hill, was a method for turning the world into a laboratory. A chemist at a bench could control all the factors affecting his experiment, altering a single one at a time and thereby learning its effects. Doctors were faced with situations in which an infinite number of influences were always colliding. Statistics was simply a way of teasing them apart. Given the wild and wilful nature of the world, analysing numbers was the only way to understand great expanses of it.

Take control groups, for example. 'The essence of the problem in a simple experiment is . . . to ensure beforehand that, as far as is possible, the control and treated groups are the same in all *relevant* respects.' Hill's emphasis drew attention to the difficulty. No matter what your suspicions, you could never know for certain all the important factors that were going to predict your patient's response to a therapy. You might carefully match your controls with respect to age or height or weight, but could you ever be sure that they were identical in every way that mattered? Even if you were, there was always the possibility of differences between them that were inconceivable to you, that were unforeseen. That meant your control group might always be crucially ill-matched. For pulmonary tuberculosis, it might be that the people whose lungs you collapsed were already fated, in some hidden way, to do better than those you left alone. Cause and effect got too easily muddled up.

This was a problem that Francis Galton had touched upon. Half seriously, but with his characteristic ingenuity, he had once tried to apply statistical methods to investigating the power of prayer. The liturgy of the Church of England included prayers for the long life of the nobility. The higher up the aristocrat, the more churchgoers would be praying for their continued survival. At the top of the tree, prayed for by more people than any of those beneath them, were the kings and queens. Yet they lived, Galton noted, shorter lives than any of the other aristocrats – shorter even than army officers, artists, writers and scientists, people for whom virtually no one thought to pray. It seemed as though prayer had no effect whatsoever. The possibility remained, however, that aristocratic prestige went along with grave and ascending ill-health, and that without those masses of prayers the royal family and others might have lived even shorter lives. Just from the association of two observations, there was no way of working out for certain if one caused the other.

So Hill was aware that a statistical association was not the same as a demonstration of causality, and that no control group could ever be matched with perfect precision for every possible factor. Doctors objected that these problems meant the utility of statistics was a foolish illusion; expert opinion might be flawed, but it was less flawed than the alternatives.

Not true, said Hill. Differentiating causation from association was possible if you intervened rather than simply observed. Or at least it was possible if you could solve the problem of matching two groups of people with enough confidence to be sure that they were effectively identical. That is, if you could find two groups who were *exactly* the same as one another, in every imaginable and unimaginable way, then you could do something to one of them and not to the other. Any resulting difference between the two would then be definitely due to your intervention. But how could two people ever be found who were identical? Even in the womb, twins that share exactly the same genes already begin to have different experiences. No two people were ever precisely the same.

What Hill proposed in his *Lancet* articles and in his book, was 'the allocation of alternate cases'. As in the trial of horse serum for treating pneumonia, you could take one person and put them in one group, then place whoever came next in the other group. Given enough people, all differences would balance out. The glory of the method was that the differences would balance *regardless* of whether you knew about them or not. Here was the answer to the problem, the method that could produce groups of people that were identical not only in the ways you knew about, but also the ones you didn't know. Of course you could never guarantee *completely* that the groups matched, but you could get close. Flip a coin a thousand times in a row and there is a chance it will always come up heads. The more times you flip, though, the more confident you can be that heads and tails will – on average – spread themselves evenly.

Within Hill's writing, though, were some notable omissions. As an example of the effects of alternate allocation, Hill presented data from the MRC's trial of serum therapy for pneumonia. In one very obvious respect, the matching was clearly a failure. Young patients were more likely to have got the serum, older ones more likely not to. Given that the older you were, the more fatal pneumonia became, that was a problem. Hill did not comment on how it was that the two groups of men came to differ; the implication was that the trial had simply been too small to smooth the groups into similarity. It included only 322 patients. Hill noted that 159 had been controls, and 163 had been treated with the serum. He did not remark that there was something wrong with those numbers. If the patients were really being allocated alternately, to one group and then another, then the total of 322 should have divided equally down the middle. It didn't.

There was only one explanation, and Hill did not mention it. The doctors had cheated. The alternate allocation was a failure because the doctors could influence it. A hunch that this person should get the serum, or that another should not, and the trial had become compromised. There was always an urge to do as much as possible for the youngest patients. Doctors were unable to resist the temptation to try to help. It seemed that if there was a way for doctors to influence which patients got which therapies, they did so. Picking different sorts of people for the different options meant that the results of the trial became meaningless. It was not badly intentioned, it was not something Hill was incapable of sympathising with, but it was a problem all the same. Overcoming it was the one thing that Hill's book did not discuss.

As a boy, Ronald Aylmer Fisher was uncertain whether to follow his interests in biology or in mathematics. According to his Royal Society memoir, the decision was made when he saw a museum display of a cod. The bones of the fish's skull were separated out and neatly labelled. Fisher promptly chose maths.

At Cambridge, he came across the work of Karl Pearson. It influenced him greatly, although the two men later fell out over a statistical concept known as likelihood ratios. When the First World War broke out, Fisher tried to join the army. They rejected him, saying his eyesight was too poor. His work on statistics therefore continued. It brought him acclaim and, from Pearson, the offer of a job. Sensing the beginnings of what was to become a lifelong feud, Fisher turned him down. His interest in identifying problems that required mathematical solutions continued. 'A lady declares that by tasting a cup of tea made with milk she can discriminate whether the milk or the tea infusion was first added to the cup,' he wrote in 1935. 'We will consider the problem of designing an experiment by means of which this assertion can be tested.'

Working in an agricultural research institute, he applied himself to studying the way in which statistics could most reliably aid scientific discovery. What he came up with was one of the most important, as well the most obscurely obvious, ideas in human history: namely that in certain circumstances, 'only randomisation can provide valid tests of significance'.

Scientific method does not just mean doing *a* test. It means doing a *reliable* test. Without that, all the trappings of an experiment are a lie, a way for people to convince themselves and others that they possess something truthful when they do not. Fisher figured out the step that was missing from Hill's explanation of trial design. Alternate allocation simply was not robust enough to make sure that two groups matched each other.

Fisher was not thinking of patients but of plots of ground. His agricultural research was aimed at replacing myths with facts. How could you figure out what actually worked? No two fields were ever quite the same and it was never entirely possible to pick out two groups of plots that perfectly matched. They varied like people did, both in ways you could see and measure and also in ones you could not. But if you took enough fields, and allocated them at random, then everything should balance out. Your tests should work, your science should be reliable and the conclusions you reached as helpful as the truth could possibly be.

Stirred by the commercial success of streptomycin in America, British drug companies were gearing up to produce it themselves. Until they did so, supplies were exceedingly limited. America was willing to export a certain amount of the drug to Britain. Fifty kilos was a substantial quantity, but it was limited all the same. It came at the hefty price, in 1946, of a third of a million dollars.

Reading accounts of what happened next, you can get the impression that doctors did the only thing they could with the quantity of drug available to them. With tuberculosis such a common disease, fifty kilos (110 pounds) was nowhere near enough to treat everyone suffering from it. The Medical Research Council decided that the drug should be given with reasonable freedom to those afflicted by rapidly fatal forms of tuberculosis, like the meningitis it produced when it got into the coverings of the brain. Those people were an unfortunate minority. For them, any outcome other than death would be proof that the new drug worked – and side effects were not an issue.

The bulk of tuberculosis, though, was a different thing. Doctors knew that many people were likely to recover without streptomycin, and that they often made full recoveries. For such patients, side effects mattered very much. And since lots of people recovered from tuberculosis without any help, it was difficult to determine how much difference the drug made. The Medical Research Council described its actions as though there was only one possible course of action: a well-organised trial.

Today, that would be true. In 1946 it was propaganda. The streptomycin could easily have been sold on the open market, or distributed evenly for doctors to use as they saw fit. Those were the normal processes; that was how America was behaving. Part of the reason that the MRC took such care to make it seem that a trial was the only way forward was because it needed to persuade people who still found the idea of trials repugnant. It was not just trying to establish the effects of a new drug; it was trying to set a precedent.

The MRC's trial of streptomycin was revolutionary.* It was not a revolution that the wider community of doctors had looked for. They were still too reliant on their self-confidence, too little affected by the small amount of statistical theory they knew. The Medical Research Council, however, found itself in a position to bully doctors into behaving as it thought best. Since a 1911 Act of Parliament, the care of tuberculous patients had been put in the hands of local authorities. That centralised the control of therapies to a helpful degree. Now this drug was being imported in a limited amount, all of which was going to be controlled by the MRC. If doctors wanted to get hold of it for their patients, they needed to do as they were told. There was going to be no room for those who decided they did not believe in control groups, or thought they possessed the skill to predict the drug's actions without participating in a reliable experiment. The council's committee was perfectly familiar with the fact that many tuberculous therapies turned out to be useless or harmful. It knew about Sanocrysin, and understood its lesson.

Between January and September 1947, 109 patients were recruited into the MRC's trial of streptomycin for pulmonary tuberculosis. Using a prearranged list of random allocations, fifty-five patients were assigned to get streptomycin. Another fifty-two got what was

* A much abused word. Originally it meant an upheaval that returned the world to the way it was to begin with, the way it was supposed to be, to an Eden before the Fall. Here, for once, the original sense is accurate. Throughout history, medicine was supposed to be providing treatments that helped people. For almost all of that time it was failing to do so. Now the MRC was going to make absolutely sure that it understood streptomycin well enough to use it only for good. Medicine was going to be returned, not to what it had actually been, but to what it was always meant to be.

believed to be the best alternative treatment – bed-rest in a specialist TB sanatorium. Two others died within a week of joining the trial, before they could be allocated to either group.

As much as possible, in order to stop people's expectations affecting the outcomes, the existence of the trial was kept secret. Neither the patients receiving the streptomycin nor those getting the bed-rest were told of what was going on. For the latter, no fake drug was administered. The MRC knew that this was a potential problem, and understood that the placebo effect of being hospitalised might not be the same as that of being hospitalised and injected. Streptomycin, however, was given in four painful injections a day, not into a vein but deep into a muscle, and those injections were repeated for months. It would have made the groups more similar to inject water into the controls, but it was agreed that the difference was unlikely to matter enough to inflict this on people.

After six months of the trial, doctors found that there were still tubercle bacilli in the majority of patients, whether they were getting the streptomycin or not. More encouragingly, though, death rates differed markedly between the two groups of patients. Fourteen of the controls were dead; only four of those on the antibiotic. 'The difference between the two series is statistically significant,' reported the trialists. They explained their calculation. The probability of the difference having occurred by chance alone was less than one in a hundred.

The eventual effects of streptomycin turned out to be reasonably complicated. Tuberculosis, even in an individual patient, quickly grew drug resistant. That meant that although the benefits were real, the drug actually performed badly if given by itself as a cure for the disease. (In the six months after the trial finished, nine more of the control patients died – but this time the number of deaths in the streptomycin group was eight, no longer a significant difference.)

In some ways, the MRC trial of streptomycin was less innovative than it appeared. Ideas about using controls and randomisation were spreading, and not just in medicine. Their successful use was going to come; this just happened to be the trial that brought it in sooner rather than later. It was not quite even the first medical trial to make full use of this new technique of randomisation. Another MRC trial, also involving Hill, was under way on whooping cough vaccines, but the streptomycin trial was the first one to be finished and reported.

Nor was the bureaucracy that made the trial possible entirely new. The increasing power of central groups of doctors and other researchers had been growing for a while. Industrialisation, the cost of drugs, the emergence of state-run health care services, all of these things combined to make it easier for the MRC to have its way. 'As in numerous other contemporary projects,' commented Richard Doll, 'such as the wartime penicillin studies in the United States, central control enabled researchers to follow their methodological predispositions.' And that made all the difference.

Towards the end of his life, Austin Bradford Hill revealed the reason that his book and articles spoke only about alternate allocation. His initial omission of the concept of randomisation was straightforward, and deliberate. The talk of allocating a patient randomly, Hill believed at the time, was simply too much for doctors to cope with. He suspected it would scare them off completely, at least until a trial demonstrating its usefulness could be forced upon them. 'There were too few physicians,' wrote Doll, 'leave alone surgeons, who were willing to expose their theories to cold scientific investigation.'

A shortage of streptomycin, and a concentration of power, made the MRC's trend-setting trial possible. But it also came about because of a small number of people were convinced that statistical methods were the only way of telling pharmacology from fantasy. Their persuasiveness meant that medicine based on reliable evidence – not rumour, impression and intuition – began to take hold. That, more than streptomycin, was the most successful blow struck against tuberculosis. Other new antibiotics were soon developed, and they were tested and retested until combinations were found that showed the greatest likelihood of destroying the bug and leaving the patient unharmed.

Tuberculosis used to be called the Captain of the Men of Death. It seemed that way. It was to be seen everywhere, striking people down at will: the old and the young, the strong and the feeble, the rich and poor. The traditional treatments were useless. Koch did something tremendous when he discovered the tubercle bacillus, revealing it to the world and to the astonished Paul Ehrlich. The development of the randomised controlled trial, less heralded, was more important.

Statistics has remained a generally unpopular discipline, unappealing by virtue of its technicalities and its sums. It can be a difficult field, easy to get lost in and vulnerable to mistakes and misunderstandings as well as deliberate misuse. The value of it, however, is real. Numbers might be cold and critical, but the benefits they offer can be warm, compassionate and humane.

Particularly in journalism, statistics are used in such meaningless ways that people are encouraged to see them all as worthless and even dishonest. Numerators without denominators, inappropriate comparisons, a general fuzziness about where a number comes from or what it actually means: all of these things devalue statistics. Certain questions about the world, however, require a numerical approach. In medicine, where many of these questions arise, arriving at a wrong answer means people suffer and die – and the alternative to counting is relying on a guess.

17   Ethics and a Glimpse of the Future

When it published the results of the streptomycin trial in 1948, the Medical Research Council was on the offensive. The earlier results of the drug in America, it noted, were promising but inconclusive. So many people got better from TB anyway that it was difficult to tell if a new drug worked. The previous history of drug treatment for the disease, it pointed out, was catastrophic – 'The exaggerated claims made for gold treatment [Sanocrysin], persisting over 15 years, provide a spectacular example.'

Something that troubled the MRC team, and that it suspected would trouble its readers in the *British Medical Journal*, was the fact that it chose not to treat some patients. The existence of an untreated control group was controversial. To an extent, the sheer limitations of the streptomycin supply provided a neat excuse. The team could fall back on claiming that there was not enough of the drug to go around anyway. Given the situation, said Hill, 'it would have been unethical not to have seized the opportunity to design a strictly controlled trial which could speedily and effectively reveal the value of the treatment'.

The fact that it had only fifty kilos of streptomycin was true enough, but this was also dodging the issue, and the team knew it. Here was a radically effective new way of exploring whether a treatment worked. The MRC wanted to encourage other trials of the same nature, whether its members were testing drugs that were in limited or even in plentiful supply. Untreated controls were an essential part of their method.

What did the doctors involved really think about deliberately not treating half of their patients? They could have argued, using the example of Sanocrysin, that streptomycin was as likely to be harmful as to be helpful. On that basis, not treating people was as ethically reasonable as treating them. During the trial, however, a senior MRC doctor fell ill with pulmonary tuberculosis. If his colleagues really felt unsure about the qualities of the new drug, they could have encouraged him to enter the trial, like the other patients, and to take his chances. Instead, the MRC arranged for their doctor to receive streptomycin. They treated him outside the trial, so as not to bias its results with the entry of a patient who had no wish to be randomised, but they treated him all the same.

There was a general feeling that the drug was likely to help. The doctors behaved towards their patients in one manner and towards themselves in another.

On Christmas Eve 1947, Eric Arthur Blair was admitted to hospital with pulmonary tuberculosis. Since meeting Cochrane during the Spanish Civil War, Blair had become famous under his adopted name of George Orwell. Two months after his admission, in the midst of a Scottish February, he wrote to his publisher about his doctor's plans to give him 'some new American drug called streptomycin'.

It took some doing, since Orwell was not part of the MRC trial. It involved buying the drug directly in America, with dollars earned from Orwell's *Animal Farm*. Even then there were problems: the US export restrictions, and the British Board of Trade. Orwell, though, was well connected. His publishers were influential people, and Aneurin Bevan, the Labour Minister for Health, was a previous editor of his journalism. The drug soon arrived. Orwell became the first man in Scotland to get it. To begin with, it made him feel better. Then things changed:

> ... my face became noticeably redder & the skin had a tendency to flake off, & a sort of rash appeared all over my body, especially down my back ... It was very painful to swallow & I had to have a special diet for some weeks. There was now ulceration with blisters in my throat & in the insides of my cheeks, & the blood kept coming up into little blisters on my lips. At night these burst & bled considerably, so that in the morning my lips were always stuck together with blood & I had to bathe them before I could open my mouth. (Bastian, 2004)

Orwell's hair and nails fell out. Like the bleeding and the rash, this seemed to be a reaction to the streptomycin. Orwell wrote to a friend, coining his own image to express the delicate balance his doctors were trying to find between streptomycin's benefits and harms: 'I suppose with all these drugs,' he said, 'it's rather a case of sinking the ship to get rid of the rats.'

As his reaction grew worse, streptomycin was withdrawn. Most of the side effects soon faded, although Orwell's nails never properly grew back. He was kept in hospital, prevented from spending time with his son and even – such were the demands of the prescribed bed-rest – prevented from writing. Desperate to finish his novel *1984*, he tore his way through it, closing his life with the feeling that the rush and the sickness caused him to ruin it. 'I ballsed it up rather,' he concluded. The misery of feeling he had botched his book did not get rid of his urge to try and do something better: 'I must try and stay alive for a while because apart from other considerations I have a good idea for a novel.'

Orwell died in January 1950. The final part of his life was destroyed partly by the side effects of streptomycin, which the MRC trial made clear was the flip-side of a generally beneficial drug, but also by the needless bed-rest – which was, in contrast, an entirely avoidable and pointless harm. Truth is corruptible – that was one of the messages of Orwell's *1984*. It is vulnerable, but so long as people cling to numbers, so long as they insist that two plus two make four, it can be protected. Opinions and propaganda are capable of distorting the world but numbers are not so easily swayed.

The Medical Research Council's work, the culmination of a long historical rise in statistical thinking, showed something similar. The randomised controlled trial could sweep away the propaganda of drug companies wanting to sell expensive products, of eminent physicians blinded by their own self-belief, of doctors misled by good intentions and the play of chance. For the first time, doctors had a way of reliably discovering the truth about the world.

It gave rise to new problems. In his *Principles of Medical Statistics*, Austin Bradford Hill raised two questions that troubled him. 'It is impossible to ignore the fact that in the random allocation of patients to the treated and untreated categories,' he noted, 'a difficult moral issue is often raised. The treatment is usually based on a priori evidence which suggests that it should have some curative effect. Can it, then, be justifiably withheld from any patient? And if it is withheld how extensive a trial is justifiable?' Hill might have added a third question, too: 'What sort of people should be randomly allocated to experimental trials, and what sort immediately given the newest and most promising treatment available?'

It was clear that the role of statistics was fundamental to medical research. If you wanted to know if something cured or killed, you had to be in the business of counting. If everyone who took it immediately dropped dead, coming to a conclusion was easy. If the difference was smaller then you needed to be more sophisticated. That meant thinking about statistics from the very beginning. You could not blunder your way thoughtlessly to begin with, then use some sort of statistical analysis to sort yourself out afterwards. Statistics needed to be part of your plan from the start.

Karl Pearson's argument for randomisation was actually quite different from Hill's. Pearson distrusted other techniques, fearing that they would not sufficiently spread traits across the groups being compared – Hill, on the other hand, just distrusted the doctors. His feeling was that they were simply unable to let go of their belief that they knew, in advance of a trial, which treatment was best. The experience of the MRC serum study, like the weight of thousands of years of medical history before it, appeared to prove him right.

It was also true, as Hill was clearly aware, that these statistical techniques offered problems as well as solutions. Not only were they technically demanding, but they had emotional costs too. Going along with a randomised controlled trial meant summoning up the humility to put your ideas to the test, and designing experiments that were capable – despite how much you believed something was going to turn out true – of proving you wrong. Hill summed up what he expected doctors to screw themselves up into doing: 'The more anxious we are to prove that a difference between groups is the result of some particular action we have taken or observed, the more exhaustive should be our search for an alternative and equally reasonable explanation of how that difference has arisen.' That was the essence of the new medicine's hard-won scepticism.

Beyond it, there were the ethical problems, ones that Hill had more difficulty in resolving. Unleashing a medicine without under-standing its effects was clearly irresponsible. What about only giving it to half the people asking for it, though, because you are insisting on running a trial? Was that not also wrong? What about those people in the control group? The answers were not clear, but the alternatives were. Small and badly designed trials could too easily give the wrong answers. Life-saving treatments got abandoned as a result, and others that caused suffering and death were mistakenly adopted in their place. There were real moral difficulties about withholding a new treatment from half of those who might benefit, but was not giving an untested drug outside of a trial morally worse? It certainly held out the prospect of harming far greater numbers of people. As relying on therapeutic hunches had failed for millennia, there was no reason to think it was suddenly going to start becoming a successful strategy now.

Giving a drug outside of a trial not only meant that lost benefits and added harms were potentially vaster, it also meant they had no hope of coming to an end. Without a trial, the answer might never be known. Was it not at least better to give the wrong treatment to half of a small group of people, for a limited time, in the expectation of learning from the experience? Rather than just guessing and risking giving the wrong treatment to everyone for evermore?

John Crofton was a junior doctor involved in running the MRC trial of streptomycin. Almost sixty years later, he wrote an account of his experiences. His feeling for the importance of the study comes across. Streptomycin's role in tuberculosis became rapidly understood in a way that was impossible through any other method. And the precedent set by the trial was superb. Crofton noted that 'when Archie Cochrane was pondering which of the specialities within medicine had made most determined efforts to base policies and practices on the results of reliable research he had no hesitation in awarding the "gold medal" to the tuberculosis specialists'. Having seen the power of trials to illuminate their own field, these doctors were more persuaded than many of their colleagues. Crofton himself went on to be part of a group that showed bed-rest to do more harm than good. Across the world, the sanatoria were closed.

Despite all this, Crofton made two revealing and surprising remarks. 'Randomised trials like these', he said of the streptomycin one, 'were of great practical importance in developing effective treatment strategies, but they were not intellectually challenging.' He knew he was making history with the streptomycin trial, and he still found something about it boring.

Then, right at the end of his reminiscences, Crofton recalls the many doctors from Britain and abroad who later came to visit his hospital. The great majority, he remembered, were interested in what his trials had found – not the methods by which they found them. You could set the best precedent in the world, and most of the medical profession was not going to be interested. Getting doctors to pay attention to results was straightforward; making them think about methods was torture.

Running a trial involved a lot of forms, a lot of protocol, and a lot of time. It was dull, it was methodical. The actual performance of it gave doctors no opportunity to enjoy the decision-making and intellectual effort that they normally relied on for job satisfaction. It couldn't: the whole point of the trial was to temporarily remove the ability of individual doctors to make decisions. That was what you needed to do in order to see what happened when people were treated according to a strict protocol.

Methodical tests remain something that most doctors do not enjoy: an ongoing problem when it comes to doing them, and a clue as to why they took so long to develop in the first place. Their effects have been unmistakable all the same. 'The Medical Research Council's trials were designed according to statistical analyses made by Bradford Hill and, later, by Ian Sutherland,' concluded the scientist Max Perutz:

They have been crucial to the near-eradication of tuberculosis in developed and many underdeveloped countries throughout the world. They were the first to evaluate the efficacy of treatments free from human bias and according to rigorous mathematical criteria, and they have helped to transform clinical practice from an art into a science.

Archie Cochrane played no part in the MRC streptomycin trial, but it affected him profoundly, as he recorded in his memoir:

> It was at this time that I began to wonder and discuss with my colleagues how other forms of medical treatment would stand up to the test of the randomised controlled trial. Looking back, this is undoubtedly the point at which the immense potential of [it] . . . began to dawn on me. It offered clinical medicine, and health services generally, an experimental approach to questions of effectiveness and efficiency, and a massive step forward from 'validation' by clinical opinion and essentially subjective observations. I think it was the simplicity of the idea in relation to the magnitude of the advance it represented that captured my imagination.

Enthralled, Cochrane was one of the minority able to take intellectual delight in the opportunities this approach offered, and the doubts it cast on the benefits of expert opinion – something he was habitually sceptical about. Most of his work was on the lung diseases of Welsh miners, their causes and treatments, and the ways in which doctors could most usefully gather and think about the relevant information. He made a few forays into other areas. Cardiologists become a favourite target. Electrocardiograms are recordings of the heart's electrical activity, the jagged lines so beloved of TV and film directors. Cardiologists claim skills in reading them that are beyond the measure of other doctors. Cochrane took randomly selected ECGs and sent copies to four different senior cardiologists, asking them what the tracings showed. He compared their opinions and found that these experts agreed only 3 per cent of the time. Their confidence in being able to look at the tracings and see the 'truth' did not seem justified. At least ninety-seven times out of a hundred, someone was getting something wrong. When Cochrane performed a similar test with professors of dentistry, asking them to evaluate the same mouths, he found that there was only a single thing that their diagnostic skills consistently agreed on: the number of teeth.

Convinced of the uselessness of most untested medical opinions, Cochrane was willing to take what appeared, to other doctors, to be risks. During a routine screening as part of his research, he found one man, 'a very likeable, cheerful, tough young miner, married with two children', whose chest X-ray showed lymphoma, a type of cancer. The man felt completely well. The accepted treatment was immediate radiotherapy. The side effects were known to be crippling, and no tests had ever been done to prove the widespread medical prejudgement that they were worthwhile. Cochrane decided not to tell the man, to 'protect' him from what the cancer specialists believed, without evidence, to be life-prolonging treatment. Instead he arranged for the man's family doctor to follow him up surreptitiously. 'He lived happily for another 10 years. He paid off his mortgage and had another child. I felt justified. He died rapidly after developing symptoms.'

In 1956 a surgeon removed a swollen gland from Cochrane's armpit. It was meant to be a routine procedure, but when he woke from the operation Cochrane found his chest wrapped in vast swathes of bandages. 'I must tell you the truth,' the surgeon said, coming into the room soon after and looking grave. 'Your axilla [armpit] is full of cancerous tissue.' He explained to Cochrane that it seemed the cancer was advanced and inoperable. There was probably little time left.

The surgeon made his decision about the nature of Cochrane's disease on the basis of what he saw on opening him up. The normal procedure, if there was any doubt about the appearance of a lump during an operation, was to have a piece of it examined immediately under a microscope by a pathologist. The surgeon was certain enough of his judgement to make that unnecessary. Trusting his own opinion, he had not stopped at cutting away the original gland, but had gone on to remove a large part of Cochrane's chest wall and the attached muscles.

Cochrane lay in his bed planning how he should spent his last days, and thinking of where it was that he wanted to be when he died. For all his scepticism, when he was on the receiving end of such a serious medical opinion, he trusted the professional skills of his colleagues. The tissue cut out of him had not yet been fully examined, but he accepted that the diagnosis was certain. 'I had been told that the pathologist had not yet reported, but I never doubted the surgeon's words.'

The gland turned out not to contain any cancer at all; the surgeon's impression of his own infallibility was a fiction. It was yet another lesson for Cochrane of the dangers of doctors who think too much of their own opinions. Restored to vigorous scepticism, and to equally good health, Cochrane continued his personal campaign to persuade people that whatever could be tested, should be tested. As a Cambridge medical student he had laboured to learn the detailed anatomy required of him; his efforts placed him first in his year. They were probably, he thought in retrospect, completely useless. What was the point of cramming incredibly intricate anatomical knowledge into medical students at the beginning of their courses? He suggested they should be tested, a few years later, to see if any of them remembered enough of it to justify the high opinion that their teachers placed on their efforts. The Professor of Anatomy, convinced without any such evidence that these early labours were good for the students, refused to co-operate.

When two different ways of running the local medical school were suggested, Cochrane suggested that, rather than trusting to their mutual ability to recognise the best one, they perform a trial. He suggested adopting one method at Cardiff and the other at nearby Bristol. Then they could allocate students, most of whom applied to both, randomly to one of the two schools. In a few years' time they would be able to objectively see which system produced the best results. His colleagues laughed.

Having been beaten as a schoolboy, Cochrane wondered whether different forms of punishment in prisons and schools might be tested. 'Corporal punishment had made an impression on me . . . Since then I had often wondered about the value of such "correction", which so many extolled and yet so few had sought to validate.' He tried and failed to find any schools willing to co-operate. He had no success at getting the government to test prison policies, reporting that 'civil servants have consistently exhibited hysterical reactions to the mention of randomised controlled trials'. The Conservative Party's 1979 suggestion that criminals needed a 'short, sharp, shock', Cochrane pointed out, could be tested.

> I discussed the problem privately with a number of magistrates I knew. I suggested to them the value of controlled trials, but was horrified when they reacted like elderly physicians and headmasters. They too suffered from the God complex. They knew what to do without the help of any trials. It was depressing.

Then it was back to trying to irritate cardiologists out of their settled complacency. Cochrane was concerned at the introduction of coronary care units (CCUs) in hospitals. Miniature intensive care wards, designed to look after patients brought into hospital with heart attacks, they were new and expensive and theoretically excellent. Cochrane wondered if they actually delivered anything of value. Could they conceivably make things worse? He thought it was worth checking. Perhaps the noise and machinery in them, the awareness of being monitored so intensively, made people anxious – and perhaps that anxiety was an unhealthy thing for those whose hearts were unstable. Even if the units did not harm their patients, they took a lot of NHS money away from other areas, so merely assuming that they delivered sufficient benefits to make them worthwhile was not, argued Cochrane, a good enough way to proceed.

To his amazement, the government and the Medical Research Council agreed to set up a committee to look into whether a trial might be needed. The cardiologists said it was not. They presented evidence showing that in-patient death rates from heart attacks promptly declined whenever a hospital set up one of these new CCUs. Cochrane objected that whenever a unit was opened many of the healthiest patients, who would previously have been sent straight home, ended up being admitted. That resulted in the overall inpatient population becoming very much fitter. Was it then any surprise to find that a smaller percentage of them were dying? As with Galton's investigation of prayer, an observational study could not distinguish what was cause and what was effect.

The committee was convinced, and approved a trial. The cardiologists responded by refusing to be involved in it, or let their patients near it. 'Later I became fascinated by the psychology under-lying the decision,' wrote Cochrane. 'The consultants whom I knew personally were ordinary, reasonable, intelligent people. They knew that the Platt committee had completely outflanked them intellec-tually and ethically, but they still felt a sacred right to treat patients as they wished. I was horrified.'

Cochrane eventually found some cardiologists willing to help, although he was amused to note their reasons. They were not going along with the trial because they felt their beliefs needed testing, but out of the conviction that the results would confirm their views and strengthen their arguments for more of the new units. Six months later, the committee sat again. This time the aim was to look at the data that the trial had gathered up to that point, comparing the death rates of patients randomly allocated to CCUs with those randomly selected to be sent home. Cochrane, presenting the data, knew that it showed an advantage for those patients who were sent home. It was too small, however, to be reliable – given the small numbers of patients then in the trial, it could too easily be down to luck.

Outside the committee room he showed the data to a group of the cardiologists. What he offered them, however, were not the real results, which he knew they would correctly judge to be unreliable and inconclusive. Instead he gave them a report where the number of deaths had been reversed. Rather than showing a trivial advantage to patients who were sent home, now it showed that the advantage came with being kept in a CCU. Instead of recognising the flipped data as being equally inconclusive, the cardiologists leapt on them as proof of their argument. 'They were vociferous in their abuse: "Archie," they said, "we always thought you were unethical. You must stop the trial at once . . ."' They wanted it halted because they were convinced that it was unfair to deny CCU care to any of the patients. 'I let them have their say for some time and then apologised and gave them the true results, challenging them to say, as vehemently, that coronary care units should be stopped immediately. There was dead silence.'

Later, whenever he lectured about that particular study, Cochrane found that he was always asked the same question. Despite it all, doctors wanted to know, wouldn't he himself go into a coronary care unit in the event of having a heart attack? The eventual results of the trial reflected those at the interim meeting: a statistically non-significant advantage for those treated at home. The most reasonable interpretation was to say that the two approaches were similar, the next most likely that the CCUs harmed people but the trial had not been big enough to prove it. On average, the new CCUs offered no advantages whatsoever at a very significant cost.

It gave Cochrane some pleasure to point out to his audiences that he had already made plans for his own heart attack, discussing it with his own doctor and asking to be treated at home. When he finally suffered one, during Christmas of 1981, that was exactly what happened.

The point of all of these experiences is not to show that doctors were still making mistakes. It is to demonstrate that they were still making the *same* mistakes. The surgeon who cut out the gland from Cochrane's armpit was more effective than his Egyptian predecessors of three to four thousand years before. He could provide significantly more effective care for the majority of his patients. His mentality, however, was unchanged. He was more useful than Imhotep, Hippocrates or Galen, but that was due to developments in technology provided for him by others. His method of thinking was no more advanced than his ancient predecessors. Cochrane's experience of doctors, before and after the Second World War, was of men (and increasingly of women) so possessed with faith in their own powers of perception that their potential for making mistakes and overestimating themselves was exactly that of their forebears in Sumer and Thermopylae. What Cochrane called 'the God complex' was still in place. Medicine had advanced: medics, for the most part, had not.

Towards the end of Cochrane's life, his love of his work flared up. Between the dark hours of ten in the evening and one in the morning, in his bachelor farmhouse, he sat at his desk and wrote a short book that changed the medical world. *Effectiveness & Efficiency* did what Austin Bradford Hill had not thought possible. The success of the streptomycin trial had shoved doctors' noses into evidence-based medicine against their will. Hill had described how impossible he thought it was to persuade them to wake up to the shortcomings of their intuitions and clinical judgements. His solution had been to infiltrate the Medical Research Council, to push medics into something against their wishes and fundamentally without their full knowledge and free consent. By contrast, *Effectiveness & Efficiency*, in under a hundred pages of passionate argument, demanded that those who read it held themselves up to higher standards, that mental honesty and personal integrity be allowed to prompt them into growing up and abandoning their childish beliefs in their powers of figuring out the world without method or numbers. A love of truth and a desire to help, said Cochrane's book, were required for those who wanted to understand the world and improve it. Just as he had shamed the German prison guards into properly looking after their inmates, demanding they live up to their country's better examples, now Cochrane did something similar for doctors in general.

In September 1983, his health fading, frightened that he might lose his mind to dementia, Cochrane wrote his own obituary. He mentioned porphyria, the genetic disease that affected many in his family and, certainly, in later life, himself. He also noted the medical profession's refusal to award him the financial bonus that the NHS provided to eminent or admired doctors. As he was independently wealthy, it was not the money that mattered to him. It was probably not even the recognition, only that its lack confirmed his colleagues were failing to recognise the importance of constructive scepticism, and the value of statistically thoughtful trials. 'He lived and died', said Cochrane of himself, 'a severe porphyric, who smoked too much, without the consolation of a wife, a religious belief or a merit award, but he didn't do so badly.' It seemed a fair judgement on an exceptionally well-lived and useful life.

18   Thalidomide's Ongoing Catastrophe

For as long as there have been governments and drugs there have been attempts at regulation. The desire to make sure they were enforceable limited their range. Most medical preparations were so muddled and useless that regulation of them was impossible. Beer was an ancient exception. Doctors prescribed it, patients felt its effects, brewers weighed and measured it, bureaucrats monitored its prices and its constituents. The Code of Hammurabi, named after the sixth king of Babylon, set out restrictions on beer's production and sale. Four thousand years ago, brewers who cheated their customers were thrown into the river.

Other rules came into being from the medical profession's efforts to enforce their chosen wisdoms, and protect themselves from competition. Leading doctors decreed the rightness of their methods, and the wrongness of those who argued with them. Drug purity began as an article of faith, but, like other faiths, progressively attracted an accretion of rules and approved ceremonies. The British regulatory system began in 1518, with the foundation of the Royal College of Physicians of London. It was part of the profession's attempt to retain power, prestige and central control by taking advantage of sixteenth-century bureaucracy. Setting itself up to regulate medications, as well as those using them, the college obtained the right to decide what was fit for purpose and who was allowed to practise.

Centuries later, the medical profession's modern drive for regulation was still a mix of altruism and self-interest. In 1909 and again in 1912, the British Medical Association published reports on 'Secret Remedies', prodding Parliament into setting up a committee to investigate quack medicines. The prospect of people dosing themselves with these remedies was horrifying to the doctors, even though their medically supported treatments were likely to be as bad as those available without a prescription. In addition, legislation in 1917 led to some restrictions on the way a drug could be promoted. For the first time, a company was not allowed to claim health benefits that were not generally accepted as being real – although only for products relating to sexual diseases and for cancer. Other conditions took longer.

The restrictions, however, were pretty minor, since the proof of effectiveness required was no more than a proof of opinion. The Therapeutic Substances Act in 1925 tried for something limited but objective: to guarantee that descriptions of a medicine's ingredients were accurate. By the end of the 1950s, despite this handful of measures, British systems for drug regulation were barely more advanced than those of four centuries before. The pharmaceutical industry was changed out of all resemblance to the apothecary shops of days gone by, but the legal controls were largely unaltered.

Historically, the regulation of drugs failed to provide any benefits for patients, although it protected the status and the earnings of doctors. Both groups were under the illusion that drugs were generally helpful. What regulation there was made it more likely that people were getting the goods they were paying for. That was all you could expect of it.

Accurately controlling the chemical compositions of treatments was impossible until about two hundred years ago. Only in exceptional circumstances were regulators willing to stand over people as they made something, then certify it as sound. In other situations, the lack of chemical techniques for analysing a product made it impossible to work out what was actually in it. So long as that scarcely mattered – one remedy being most likely as useless or poisonous as another – this was not an issue. But with effective drugs came effective rules. Paul Ehrlich's introduction of Salvarsan in 1910 resulted in the British Board of Trade checking on the composition of products claiming to contain it. Advances in chemistry meant that constituents were measurable, and here was something whose concentration genuinely mattered.

Consumers could not tell the purity of a drug by tasting it, nor could they accurately understand the effects of a tablet by swallowing one and seeing what happened. Without an equable distribution of knowledge, the manufacture and sale of drugs could clearly not be left to an entirely free market. The number of milligrams of an active ingredient in a pill, and the likely effects of that pill, were similar in this respect to the number of calories in a mouthful of food, or the origins of a pack of coffee. Medicines had become what economists call 'credence goods', items that an average person could not fully assess for themselves. The public had to trust those who were making and supplying them, and regulation was needed to stop that trust being abused.

Towards the end of the nineteenth century the US Department of Agriculture (USDA) had become increasingly concerned about the way products were adulterated before sale. The emerging power of chemistry gave producers an increasing ability to alter food. A series of reports from the USDA helped drive public worries about the issue. What were people adding to food in order to change its colour, weight, smell or appearance? Were these additives safe? Harvey Washington Wiley, chief chemist at the USDA from 1883, campaigned successfully to publicise these problems. His efforts were rewarded in 1906, when Theodore Roosevelt signed into law the Food and Drugs Act. Often referred to as the Wiley Act, in the chemist's honour, it gave the USDA the power and responsibility to examine food and drugs. The officials were empowered to look for evidence of cheating in the way those goods were made and sold.

Curiously, the Act did not restrict the health claims people could make for their products – only their ability to lie about ingredients. Those who wrote the Act drafted it with the intention that it should do more, but they were stopped in 1911 when the Supreme Court heard a case regarding a quack medicine – 'Dr John's Mild Combination Treatment for Cancer' – and ruled that the Act did not prevent any medical claims a manufacturer wanted to make. An amendment the following year was meant to fix the problem, adding 'false and fraudulent [claims of] curative or therapeutic effect' to the list of illegal ways of presenting a product. The courts, however, demanded that proof rest on a demonstration that someone was being intentionally false about his or her beliefs. Sincerity, in other words, was enough to justify a health claim. Accuracy of judgement was irrelevant. And insincerity was exceptionally difficult to prove in a court of law.

From 1930, the USDA's Bureau of Chemistry, now headed by Wiley's successor, became the Food and Drug Administration (FDA). In that name it was asked to respond to the after-effects of the efforts by the Massengill Company, of Bristol, Tennessee, in 1937, to produce palatable sulphonamides. Rather than a powder, Massengill wanted to sell the drug as a liquid. Their chief chemist, Harold Watkins, dissolved it in diethylene glycol, a substance very closely related to antifreeze and with many of the same properties, then added fruit syrup to make it taste pleasant. The company sold the drug without testing it on animals and without paying attention to existing knowledge about diethylene glycol's toxicity. It was on sale for a little over two months and it killed 107 people.

When the FDA arrived at Massengill's headquarters, it found the company had already realised its mistake. It had voluntarily withdrawn the drug. The notices it sent out, though, only asked for the drug to be returned – they made no mention of how dangerous it was. Only at the FDA's insistence was a second round of warnings released, this time mentioning that the drug could kill.

While the FDA co-ordinated efforts to recover the drug, Massengill's owner denied any blame. 'We have been supplying a legitimate professional demand, and not once could have foreseen the unlooked-for results.' In its way, it was a brilliant phrase. It was, indeed, impossible to foresee results that you made no efforts to look for. Massengill's chemist, Harold Watkins, was more willing to take responsibility. After reading the reports of what his drug had done, he killed himself.

Once the bodies were all buried, it turned out that Massengill's operations were almost entirely within the rules. Failing to check on diethylene glycol and failing to test their product was entirely legal. Putting a lethal ingredient into a medication broke no laws; incompetence was not a crime. Massengill bore no legal responsibility for the deaths that resulted from its actions. The company, like many others after, was happy to regard this as being the final conclusion to the matter. Responsibility was taken to be a matter of law, not morality.

There was one small rule that it had broken. The drug was marketed as an *elixir* of sulphonamide. According to law, an elixir was a liquid containing alcohol, and Massengill used diethylene glycol instead. So it was guilty of mislabelling. For this, under the 1906 Food and Drugs Act, it was fined.

Public outrage led to the passage of the 1938 Food, Drug and Cosmetic Act. It required that drug companies demonstrate proof of safety – not necessarily before using the drug on people, but at least before openly marketing it. To a small degree, it also made it legally more difficult for companies to claim unjustified health benefits. The Act was limited, however, by contemporary knowledge of what constituted evidence. Proof of safety, like proof of effectiveness, was not something that could be reliably established without randomised controlled trials – and these did not yet exist.

Twenty years later, from 1959 onwards, Senator Estes Kefauver of Tennessee began pushing for greater regulation of medicines in America. What bothered him most were the prices that drug companies were charging. The shoddy standard of proof required for safety and effectiveness was also an issue, albeit a less important and less populist one. On both fronts, however, Kefauver felt that consumers needed more protection. His efforts to provide it initially went nowhere.

At the same time, in a converted seventeenth-century copper foundry in the West German village of Stolberg, a pharmaceutical company named Chemie Grünenthal was attempting to find new drugs. Supposedly they were after antibiotics, but they invested in none of Domagk's elaborate testing systems. The company found a compound of little obvious attraction. It was not original; a Swiss firm had already tried it out and thought it worthless. The Swiss had given it to animals and seen no effect. The Germans did the same, and saw opportunity galore.

Chemie Grünenthal found that the compound did nothing what-soever to rats, mice, guinea pigs, rabbits, cats or dogs. All the animals survived. The stuff seemed almost ludicrously non-toxic. To a devoted therapeutic nihilist, this might seem a promising discovery. The placebo effect has always been powerful. Medicine in the 1950s was brimming with compounds whose harms were complacently underestimated, and whose benefits were magnified beyond their deserts. A genuinely harmless placebo, coated with the allure of modern chemistry, was potentially as good for people as it was for profits. The success of sulphonamides and penicillin, however, meant that therapeutic nihilism was out of fashion.

Two historians of Chemie Grünenthal have pointed out that the company was operating from a peculiar ethical perspective. Along with the excitement created by the discovery of antibiotics, there was also the recent experience of the Second World War. The head of research and development at Grünenthal, Heinrich Mückter, had spent the war as Medical Officer to the Superior Command of German forces occupying Krakow in Poland. His additional title was Director for the Institute of Spotted Fever and Virus Research. 'The German Army', observed the historians, 'was not renowned for missionary medical work in Poland.' The institute's title sounded to them like a euphemism for a unit conducting human experiments and researching ways of killing.

The actions of Grünenthal are difficult to make sense of. One of their chemists thought that their compound was structurally similar to barbiturates, the fabulously successful but dangerous sleeping tablets. It was true that a safer sedative could promise riches as well as human benefits, but then the drug did nothing to sedate any of the animals it had been given to. Grünenthal had a drug whose primary virtue was its inactivity. Whether from some strange faith in the emerging powers of chemistry, a medieval belief in the healing abilities of any compound, or a sweeping willingness to delude people in order to take their money, Grünenthal began pushing the drug to doctors. What happened next was a clear demonstration of the weaknesses of contemporary controls on establishing the safety and effectiveness of medicines.

Before a drug was eligible for sale in West Germany, its actions needed to be shown sufficiently clearly to convince people about what it did. Normally that meant starting off with the effects of it in animal experiments, but since the drug had not shown any, that was impossible. So instead Grünenthal gave it to doctors to try out on their patients. The anecdotal reports that came back were regarded as being sufficient to establish the drug's powers. Grünenthal suggested to doctors that the drug might be useful in controlling epilepsy (a suggestion that seems to have been based, at best, on fanciful optimism). What the doctors told them in return was that the drug helped patients to sleep.

This was wonderful, given Grünenthal's desire to see their drug as being a safe version of a barbiturate. Armed with these reports, they went back to their animal experiments and managed to create one that showed an apparent effect. They put mice in a cage and recorded that they moved about a little bit less after being given the drug. It was not a recognised way of measuring a sedative, but the intention was not to hold the drug up to the highest standards of testing. The intention was to get it licensed. Performing a test is not the same thing as performing a reliable test. Not all evidence is equal. Give people sugar pills as though they are drugs and they report a range of effects and side effects. Tell them the pills are like barbiturates but safer, and you get some people coming back and saying that they slept better after taking them. Record enough different measures of an animal's movements and, eventually, one of them will correlate with whatever drug you want it to. Science, like a hammer, is only useful if you know what you are doing with it.

On Christmas Day 1956, in Stolberg where Grünenthal was based, a child was born without ears. The father had brought home drug samples from Grünenthal, where he worked, and given them to his wife during her pregnancy. Ten months later, on the first day of October 1957, three days before Sputnik took to the heavens, Grünenthal commercially released thalidomide. It spent heavily on advertising, buying space in fifty medical journals, sending out 50,000 circulars and writing directly to a quarter of a million doctors.

The drug, released under the brand name of Contergan, was a massive success. Grünenthal showed a willingness to recommend it for whatever reason people were saying they found it helpful. In 1958, after reports that it subdued vomiting, Grünenthal wrote to doctors stating it was 'the drug of choice' for treating morning sickness in pregnant women. The British company selling the drug thought this sounded like an excellent recommendation, and told their customers that thalidomide 'can be given with complete safety to pregnant women and nursing mothers, without adverse effect on mother or child'. Sales were enormous. In some countries they were second only to aspirin.

In 1959, a German neurologist wrote to Grünenthal reporting that one of his patients had developed nerve damage while taking the drug. Were they aware, he asked, of other such cases? They said no. It was a lie. Other reports were already coming in. By 1960, Grünenthal had received information describing around a hundred cases of nerve damage in people taking thalidomide. They instructed their sales representatives to deny the link, and undertook no extra research to investigate it. When their representative in Cologne was asked about thalidomide causing nerve damage, he described his response: 'I did my best to foster confusion.'

It is very hard to explain the behaviour of Grünenthal as the reports of side effects mounted. 'If I were a physician,' said Heinrich Mückter in 1961, still the company's head of research and development, 'I would not now prescribe Contergan. Gentlemen, I warn you – I do not want to repeat an earlier judgement – I see great dangers.' That was when speaking at a private company meeting. Six weeks later, at a public medical one, he described Contergan as 'the best sleeping pill in the world'.

From September the previous year, the Ohio-based company Richardson-Merrell had begun seeking approval to sell thalidomide in America. As a routine application, for a drug already accepted worldwide, the paperwork was given to the Food and Drug Administration's latest reviewer. An ex-academic, Frances Oldham Kelsey had previously worked on the fatal elixir of sulphonamide, helping to prove that it was the diethylene glycol that killed over a hundred people. She joined the FDA after a post became unexpectedly available. Her predecessor, demanding evidence of a drug's effectiveness, had abruptly lost her job – in order, it was said, 'to placate a pharmaceutical company'.

Kelsey was 'a short, slim, unpretentious woman with a sweet smile and a slight overbite'. Both her manner and her cooking were described as being rather British, an equally pejorative description whether it referred to food or to clothes. She did not seem likely to disturb the easy relationship between the drug companies and the FDA.

To the great surprise of Richardson-Merrell, Kelsey turned their application down. She was not satisfied that either the safety or the effectiveness of thalidomide was actually proven. Standards of proof were lax, but they were also barely defined. That left Kelsey free to decide on them herself. She did, and in her view the previous investigations of thalidomide did not fulfil them.

Richardson-Merrell was submitting not only thalidomide, but also an anti-cholesterol drug named MER/29. It hoped the two together would prompt its entry into 'the truly big time' of emerging American pharmaceutical companies. The anti-cholesterol drug caused blindness and other side effects in primate trials – information that the company knew about and concealed. (It was later sued by some of those damaged by the drug, paying out $200 million in compensation.) When Kelsey rejected the application, Richardson-Merrell rewrote and resubmitted it. She rejected it again, pointing out that it contained no new information. The expert opinion that supported it, thought Kelsey, was less like scientific evidence than a series of purchased testimonials.

The company grew increasingly desperate to start marketing thalidomide, directly hounding both Kelsey and her FDA superiors. At the same time, it carried on providing the drug to American doctors. FDA approval was required to market and sell a drug, but not to distribute it as part of a trial. And the proper nature of a trial was not specified. Richardson-Merrell's was not run by their researchers or pharmacists. Their trial was directed by their Sales and Marketing division. It organised the sending out of samples to doctors, reassuring them that there was no obligation to report back any results.

In Germany and Australia, doctors were already growing concerned about thalidomide. Other worries were emerging besides its ability to cause nerve damage. In the autumn of 1961 a German paediatrician named Widukind Lenz wrote to the national *Welt am Sonntag* ('World on Sunday') newspaper. He described 150 children born with severe and terrifically unusual birth defects. He linked the defects to maternal consumption of thalidomide during pregnancy. William McBride, an Australian obstetrician, wrote to the *Lancet* having reached the same conclusion in his own patients.

Lenz wrote to Grünenthal and asked them to withdraw the drug. 'Every month's delay', he wrote, 'means that fifty to one hundred horribly mutilated children will be born.' The company declined to withdraw thalidomide. Lenz's request for it to be taken off the market was followed up by one from the German government.

Later in 1961, in response to public pressure, Grünenthal withdrew the drug – although only from Germany, and only in response to what Heinrich Mückter called the 'sensationalism of the *Welt am Sonntag* story'.

A lack of records makes it impossible to accurately assess the damage caused by thalidomide. Estimates suggest that around 10,000 children were severely deformed by the drug, of whom only about half survived to be adults. In America, Richardson-Merrell's 'investigating' sales department handed out around 2.5 million tablets. It was a large number, but tiny compared to the sales elsewhere. Thanks to Kelsey's continuing refusal to approve thalidomide, fewer than twenty American children were born deformed as a result of the drug.

The pharmacologist at Grünenthal, the man whose mistake it was to believe that thalidomide resembled a barbiturate, was sickened. The thought of his drug having had such toxic effects had not occurred to him. Now it was clear what his work had led to. 'I felt like a bus driver who has run into a group of children and has killed and injured many of them,' he said.

Heinrich Mückter felt differently. When, along with eight other company executives, he faced criminal charges brought by the West German Ministry of Justice in May 1968, Mückter began with a declaration of outrage. 'I would first like to say that I still regard the charge as a gross injustice to me personally.' Chemie Grünenthal seemed to feel similarly. They fought the charges ferociously, attacking the character and the knowledge of Widukind Lenz, threatening journalists with legal action, and refusing to acknowledge any responsibility. After the third year of the trial, an out-of-court settlement of $43 million was accepted by the families of those affected. Grünenthal executives never came to judgement.

Reading the account of thalidomide on the company website you are left with the feeling that an unforeseen and unavoidable tragedy was handled with compassion and generosity by a caring corporation. Having avoided a final judgement over its legal responsibility, Grünenthal seems happy declaring itself innocent of any moral wrongdoing. The British company that sold thalidomide, Distillers, behaved in a similar manner, denying all legal and moral responsibility. Only the disgust of individual Distillers shareholders and dogged publicity in the *Sunday Times* (starting in 1972, but coming after considerable research over a ten-year period in which the British press were legally barred from discussing thalidomide) forced the company into paying compensation.

In the USA the thalidomide scandal brought Senator Kefauver's drug hearings back to life. The resulting Kefauver–Harris Amendments became law on 10 October 1962. Effectiveness and safety now needed to be proved somewhat more stringently before the FDA would license a drug. At the same time the notion of what was called 'informed consent' also passed into American law. Pharmaceutical companies were required to honestly inform people about the side effects of their products. Estes Kefauver believed that his Amendment was his 'finest achievement' when it came to keeping Americans safe.

'I do not think we need to be particularly proud', said John F. Kennedy at the time, 'that it took an international catastrophe to make us realise that the first thing with drugs is safety.' He was proud, however, of the actions he took in response. Having become President and signed Kefauver's Amendment into law, he told Congress that 'the physician and consumer should have the assurance that any drug or therapeutic device on the market today is safe *and* effective for its intended use'.

It is the sort of language that politicians are elected for using. Expressing doubt or uncertainty or caution is not the way to get into office. Kennedy's and Kefauver's confidence in the benevolence of their actions, however, was misplaced.

The point of the thalidomide story is the fragility of knowledge. What brought the drug's ill-effects to people's attention was not that it killed and maimed, but that it did so in a strikingly unusual way. It was the nature of the abnormalities that brought them to attention, not their numbers. If the deaths had been through pneumonia, or some other common disease, the fatal nature of the drug would have taken very much longer to uncover. Doctors, even the best of them, were still using drugs without the information that they needed to understand what their medicines did.

In the aftermath, this was the realisation that was missing from the world's response. Governments gave regulatory bodies new powers. The notion that medications mix an unpredictable balance of harms and benefits, whose overall sway is often not immediately apparent, was largely lost. There was very little open-minded thoughtfulness about the way in which effectiveness and safety were best assessed. Instead there was the triumphal passing of legislation.

In Germany people were struck by the fact that thalidomide was not removed by government action, or the careful compassion of pharmaceutical companies, but purely as a result of bad publicity in the press. New regulation was introduced worldwide, almost all of it following the pattern of America's FDA. Some of it helped, some made things worse.

19 Syphilis, Leprosy and Head Injuries

Albert Neisser went to school with Paul Ehrlich. Neisser, too, became a doctor, and by the time he was twenty-one, in 1878, he discovered the germ that causes gonorrhoea. A common sexually transmitted disease, without antibiotics it was capable of spreading beyond the sexual organs and causing a range of complications. It could kill. Having found its cause, Neisser went on to help discover the germ that gave rise leprosy, to found the German Society for the Fight Against Venereal Diseases, and to conduct experiments on prostitutes.

Neisser's idea was that serum therapy could be used to protect women from syphilis. He took blood from patients suffering from the disease, removed the cells and injected the remaining serum into prostitutes under his care. Some of the women whom he injected with serum later developed syphilis. Neisser concluded that his therapy had failed. When he published his findings in 1898, others added the suggestion that his serum had infected the women. The press expressed outrage. Neisser, they pointed out, had neither explained to the women what he was doing nor asked their permission.

Had Neisser's treatment worked, it would have been celebrated. Jenner is famous for having discovered the smallpox vaccine, and his human trials of it were done with exactly the same lack of consent. Neisser's therapy, however, did not work. He was fined and his actions were discussed in the Prussian parliament. A report was commissioned. It emphasised the importance of patients being fully informed about what was done to them, and being able to give or withhold their consent. In 1900 the government issued guidelines based on the report. They required 'unambiguous consent' and a 'proper explanation of the possible negative consequences' of what was proposed. The paradox was clear. If you were experimenting, you did not know exactly what an intervention's outcomes might be. That was the nature of an experiment, and it made it difficult to satisfy the demand that those participating be fully informed of all possible consequences.

By 1931, the Reich government issued clarified guidelines. Novel medical treatments required consent, 'given in a clear and undebatable manner following appropriate information'. That could be overlooked, if the situation was desperate and consent impossible – a patient unconscious and slipping towards death, for example, with no relatives available to give or refuse consent on his or her behalf.

Another problem was clearly apparent to the German authorities. Doctors had technical knowledge that patients did not. 'Informed consent' was a problematically subjective term. Patients varied immensely in the sort of information they were capable of understanding. There seemed no clear solution to this, no absolute level of comprehension required. All that was reasonable was for doctors and patients both to do the best they could; the former to explain and the latter to understand.

What was not apparent in these debates was the huge weight of inherited medical ignorance. Almost everything that doctors did, from their recommendations about diet and rest to the operations and drugs that they prescribed, had been decided on without reliable trials. As a result, only a very small proportion of what was known was actually correctly known – usually those minority of interventions that changed a situation beyond all possibility of misinterpretation. The loss of all five litres of a patient's blood, for example, was clearly accepted as fatal. The loss of half of it was still seen by some as therapeutic.

The majority of medical beliefs were guesses, yet the German government was suggesting that doctors carefully warn their patients whenever their treatment was experimental. Neither governments nor doctors could yet see that most of their treatments were worse than experimental: they were untesting, as well as untested.

Despite these failings, Germany was making creditable efforts to develop ideas about the way in which an admission of ignorance could be worked into the relationship between a doctor and a patient. It was a society with a good health care system, where the welfare state made patients confident that they would not be put in the position of having to accept openly experimental care purely because their financial means were limited. The deal was that doctors should try to be open about what they did not know, and in return recruit their patients to help them improve. A patient should be free to decide whether to agree, and whether to submit himself or herself to an unproven medical therapy.

It was also in Germany that those ideas curdled. The Nuremberg trials following the Second World War showed the extent to which doctors were eager participants – and leaders – in Nazi atrocities. Responding to the murders and vivisections carried out by Josef Mengele, Karl Brandt and others, the 1947 Nuremberg code set out ten principles for medical research. Consent was number one, and here the wording made an effort to describe what was meant by 'informed'. The consenting patient 'should have sufficient knowledge and comprehension of the elements of the subject matter involved as to enable him to make an understanding and enlightened decision'. Rather than an experimental treatment, the patient should, if they wished, be able to choose a proven one.

Two other points from the Nuremberg code are worth dwelling

on. The eighth said that 'the highest degree of skill and care should be required through all stages of the experiment'. Incompetent experiments, in other words, breach the code. The skill and care needed to get reliable results are not ornamental extras, they are essential.

The tenth point is similarly sensible, and put into words what people wished to do already. It said that those running an experiment must be willing to bring it to an end whenever they had reason to believe that continuing it was harmful. That was the principle that the cardiologists had wanted to put into action, when Cochrane gave them the false data suggesting their heart attack patients did better in hospital than at home. This point of the Nuremberg code said trials should potentially be stopped early, but added nothing at all about how certain of harm you needed to be before stopping one.

The temptation is to halt a trial the moment one treatment seems better than another. An American paediatrician, William Silverman, has pointed out that this is a bit like stopping a race the moment the horse you've backed is a nose in front. Finishing lines sometimes matter. If a trial is stopped before the difference it shows is conclusive, you can be in a worse position than before you started. Not only do you still not really know the answer, but the opportunity for finding out may be gone for good. Drugs are not ignored while evidence about them accumulates; doctors make up their minds about them regardless, wedding themselves to an opinion that it becomes very difficult to shake them out of.

From the Nuremberg code, the World Medical Association developed their 1964 Declaration of Helsinki. It has undergone five major revisions since, the last in 2000, and is intended to represent guidelines for best practice in medical research. It represents today's rough consensus. The declaration notes that research, like medical treatments themselves, must balance 'risks and burdens'. It is an impressive document, and an imposing summary of the degree to which modern medicine takes experimental method – and the ethics attached to it – seriously. When it comes to informed consent, this is what it has to say:

> In any research on human beings, each potential subject must be adequately informed of the aims, methods, sources of funding, any possible conflicts of interest, institutional affiliations of the researcher, the anticipated benefits and potential risks of the study and the discomfort it may entail.

That is an awful lot to tell to people. Its effect, like that of many of the restrictions over experimental therapies, is often destructive. Rather than always making sure that patients are kept safe, it frequently helps make sure that the necessary experiments never happen. Protecting people from the risk of trials is important. It fails to acknowledge that protecting them from the risks of treatments that have never been reliably trialled is even more so.

The later history of thalidomide remains curious. For drug companies, surprises during a drug's pre-clinical development are often full of promise. An unexpected effect can be the key to an entirely new use. Surprises during drug-testing, in contrast, are usually disastrous. The damage that thalidomide did to nerves and to embryos fell into the second category. Some doctors were astute enough, however, to realise that the drug's harmful side effects might have their own promise. Selective toxicity, the idea uncovered by Ehrlich, was a proven method of aiming a drug at a particular target. If thalidomide stopped a developing embryo from growing properly, that suggested it was toxic to cells while they were dividing. Therapies that are specifically poisonous to rapidly dividing cells are the main line of attack against cancer.

Cancerous cells are not those of a parasite. They are not like bacteria, full of molecules and receptors never found on human cells and therefore excellent targets for selective destruction. Cancer cells are our own. Mutations lead to their escaping from the normal checks and controls that the body exerts on cell division. So cells begin to grow and multiply in ways they are not supposed to. The reason so many treatments for cancer are highly toxic is that cancer cells are too similar to those around them for magic bullets to easily make a clean hit. Radiation and anti-cancer drugs are generally most harmful to cells in the process of division, since many of these will belong to the cancer. But not all. Collateral damage means that hair falls out, the lining of the gut sheds, wounds fail to heal; all those bits of the body that are constantly regenerating are harmed. The hope is that the therapy acts like the streptomycin that Orwell took for his tuberculosis. It half sinks the ship in order to get rid of the rats.

In the years immediately after thalidomide was withdrawn, three trials involving a total of around 200 people were performed in America to see if it had any promise as a cancer treatment. No useful effect was found, and interest lapsed. Then there was a piece of good fortune.

The doctor Jacob Sheskin, having fled Europe for Venezuela during the Second World War, had moved to Israel once the country was founded. He became the director of the Jerusalem Hospital for Hansen's Disease. Set up by German Protestants in the nineteenth century, it was there to look after those that others shunned. Hansen's Disease is another name for leprosy.

Leprosy is in some ways a similar disease to tuberculosis; the two germs have more than a little in common. And leprosy, like tuberculosis, can take many forms. Sheskin was looking after a man sent to him from the University of Marseilles in France. The patient was suffering from a condition called erythema nodosum leprosum. It is a form of leprosy in which the body's own antibodies, reacting with the invading organism, crystallise. These solid clumps of antibody and germ get stuck in blood vessels. They clot off the body's normal circulation. Wherever the blood has been prevented from flowing, flesh decays. Testicles, joints, bone marrow, kidneys, eyes, nerves, skin – gradually and often with a terrific amount of pain, these bits of the body have their blood choked off and begin to die. Where the circulation to a patch of skin has been cut, the skin breaks down and weeps, sections of it dying away. Boils and ulcers appear on the outside of the body. They are mirrored by similar ones, hidden and internal.

All drugs that work have side effects; anything that has an action on the human body sometimes causes unwanted reactions. The body's own responses to disease also have their own side effects. Too mild and they are not enough to keep people healthy, too fierce and the damage they do to a person's body can outweigh the harm they do to its disease. Erythema nodosum leprosum, ENL, can be an exquisitely awful way to die. It is not a manifestation of leprosy itself so much as a side effect of the body's attempt to fight it off. Even the magic bullets provided by billions of years of natural selection are not perfect.

When lots of small blood vessels clot off, they cause characteristic agony. The pain of a cramp is created by a temporary and mild failure of the body to supply enough blood. The pains of ENL are similar but worse, coming from a blood supply that is failing permanently. The man who arrived in Sheskin's Jerusalem hospital had not been able to leave his bed for almost two years. Neither sedatives nor morphine gave him more than a few moments' relief. The pain and the lack of sleep were crucifying him.

Searching for something to give him, Sheskin came across a single bottle of thalidomide pills, left forgotten in the hospital's pharmacy. Aware of their history, and remembering that they were once recommended as a sedative, Sheskin thought there was little to lose by giving them a try. Pregnancy was not a worry, and the man's nerves were already being destroyed by his disease. Thalidomide might be dangerous, but his leprosy was killing him anyway.

The effects were miraculous. Within an hour or two, the man slept properly for the first time he could remember. In the days that followed his wounds began to heal and his pain to melt away. Sheskin tried stopping the drug, and when he did so the man's symptoms returned.

Convinced that he was not witnessing a coincidence, Sheskin went on to try thalidomide with five other ENL sufferers. When they all seemed to benefit, he set up a placebo-controlled randomised trial. Published in 1965, it showed that the vast majority of ENL patients responded quickly and safely to thalidomide. (Safety, as always, is relative. The effects of the drug have to be balanced against those of the disease it treats.) A larger World Health Organisation trial went on to confirm Sheskin's results in 1971.

The main heritage that thalidomide has left us with is poisonous. Not because of what it is, but because of how it seems. Rather than a precise understanding of the dangers of flawed and insufficient evidence, we are left with a vague feeling of the general dangers of drugs. Rather than realising the essential nature of trials, we are suspicious of drug companies. Governments could have reacted to thalidomide by making sure that every drug was fully tested before being used; tested in such a way that reliable information about effects and side effects was always available. Instead they have made testing so difficult and expensive that we often do not understand the impact of the medication we take.

Thalidomide has now been found useful for some cancers. Multiple myeloma, a disease in which antibody-producing cells become cancerous, is the best example. Other benefits were found with Behçet's Disease, a rare disease of the blood vessels.

The next curious step in thalidomide's history was that people suffering from HIV found it seemed to help. It got rid of the mouth ulcers associated with their disease. In molecular terms, that was no mystery. Thalidomide seems to work in ENL (the leprosy variant) and in Behçet's by damping down inflammation – subduing the body's own response to disease, exactly as aspirin does when it eases a fever. Some of the most dangerous symptoms of HIV come when the immune system is disabled. Others, and they can be lingeringly unpleasant to live with, are due to the chronic inflammation that the disease provokes. Thalidomide can help with that. The curious part of the story was what it revealed about drug regulation.

The Food and Drug Administration is not the world's only regulatory authority, but it is America's. Any product hoping to do big worldwide business needs to comply with FDA rules. An organisation that was set up with relatively small goals – reducing adulteration of foodstuffs and the false advertising of medical remedies – now regulates a market that involves a quarter of all money spent in America. That has given the FDA unexpected power, influence, and the criticism that those things draw.

Although the FDA regulates what drugs are allowed to be sold, it has less control over the behaviour of doctors. Like its equivalents in other countries, the FDA can decide on the medical reasons that justify a drug's use. Thalidomide, it can say, is reasonable to use in order to treat ENL. What it cannot do, again like its overseas peers, is control whether doctors take any notice of it. Doctors can prescribe a drug for whatever they please. They cannot guarantee that their prescription will be honoured – that their country will sell the drug and that a nearby pharmacy will stock it – but they can prescribe it all the same. And since that means a pharmacy somewhere can make some money by honouring the prescription, then so long as the drug is legal, that is what normally happens.

In 1998 the FDA approved thalidomide for the use of leprosy patients suffering from ENL. That was a little curious, since America does not really have a problem with leprosy. But the approval meant that the pharmacies had an excuse to stock the drug. Doctors could therefore prescribe it, without paying any attention to the reasons that the FDA officially said were appropriate. The approval of thalidomide for ENL meant that American doctors could prescribe it for their AIDS patients, without any drug company having to go to the trouble of getting it approved for that use. It was a regulatory short cut, a way of avoiding the expensive trials of thalidomide in AIDS that no one was willing to fund and few people thought necessary. It appeared to be for this reason that the FDA approved the use of thalidomide for ENL.

Currently a surprising amount of prescribing is 'off-label' in this way. A 2006 survey of American physicians, published in the *Archives of Internal Medicine*, put the figure at 21 per cent. Some specialities rely on this sort of prescription more than others. Paediatricians, for example, often find that drug companies are only willing to fund trials on adults: investigating the same drugs on children is more difficult, more expensive, and not required in order to get the medications stocked by pharmacies. Once they are there, it is much easier to persuade paediatricians that the adult trials probably provide accurate predictions of how the drugs will work in children. Other minority groups, like pregnant women, are equally unattractive targets for drug trials, offering only small potential market shares. People are naturally frightened of the idea of testing drugs on children and pregnant women. What happens instead is that doctors are forced to prescribe treatments that have never been properly tested in these groups.

It seems reasonable to think that doctors should have these sorts of freedoms; more so than the drug companies trying to sell products to them. Doctors, traditionally, are trusted – the pharmaceutical industry is not. And in some ways doctors, compared to other professions, deserve the bulk of the faith that people put in them.

Money can be a factor in their behaviour, but we generally trust that intelligent compassion will be more important. It is a reasonable view, and doctors work hard to deserve it. It ignores the extent to which the sound morals of doctors have not, historically, been matched by an understanding of what they were doing. Incompetent doctors, foolish doctors and mistaken doctors can give out drugs that do not work, and prescribe therapies that harm. If someone can afterwards prove that they have acted badly, they can end up in court. But unlike the disastrous effects of thalidomide, most drug errors are not easily detectable.

There is a battle between doctors and those who want to regulate them, to control the way they behave. It is not entirely clear who should win. The doctors want to preserve their freedom over their own actions, pointing out that you need to tailor even well-justified treatments to suit particular people. What if aspirin, for example, makes them feel sick? Or they have a history of bleeding when they take it?

The other side of the argument is to point out how superbly bad most doctors are at being efficient. We know from reliable trials what drugs someone should be on if he or she is at high risk of a heart attack – aspirin, a beta blocker and a statin, for example. Surveys always show that too few people are being prescribed the medications they need. Not through any great objection on the part of their doctors, but through inefficiency. Going through checklists and ticking boxes is not something that doctors seem to be good at. (Specialist nurses, more methodical about following protocols, are often better.)

In the meantime, governments try to control doctors a little bit on the sly, through the financial rewards they give them and the way they regulate the borders of medical practice. Family doctors in Britain are now rewarded with extra money for treating certain people with certain drugs. Whenever certain prescribing practices have been tied to a reward in their wage packet, doctors appear capable of changing their behaviour greatly.

Making doctors into employees – reducing their freedoms, limiting their choices – gives governments and businesses a method of getting doctors to do what they want, a way of making them cheaper and more efficient. It offers real benefits, both for reducing the amount that a society spends on health care, and also in improving the effectiveness with which some of it is delivered. There is something horrible about the prospect of it, all the same.

The FDA has now rejected the latest revision of the Declaration of Helsinki, from 2000, objecting to two parts of it. One of the paragraphs that the agency dislikes discourages placebo trials. It suggests that new treatments should be compared with the best available alternative – being a placebo only if there isn't really anything at all.

Discouraging placebo-controlled trials can be perfectly reasonable. What doctors need to know about the latest antidepressant, antibiotic or sedative is not whether it works better than a sugar pill. They need to know how it compares to the best available treatment. Once one medication has been proven to be of benefit, all new therapies should be compared to it, not a placebo. Two active drugs, though, are likely to be more similar than one and a placebo. So trials comparing them need to be much bigger if they are going to show a difference. They need to last longer, recruit more patients, cost more. And at the moment, with the FDA's support, that is money that drug companies do not need to spend. They can take the short cut of showing that their new pill is better than a placebo, then leave it up to their marketing department to convince you (without decent proof) that it is better than its competitors.

A large amount of medical research is undertaken for marketing purposes. Since doctors still too rarely demand to see evidence that is reliable, these trials often produce enough appearance of knowledge to sway a drug's sales figures. In that they are insincere and misleading, of course, they breach the conventions put in place after the Nuremberg trials, the clauses that say that doing bad research is as much an outrage as experimenting on people against their wishes. Arguably, since it affects many more patients, bad research is worse. As medical crimes go, it is certainly more common – and it goes almost universally unpunished.

The other paragraph rejected by the FDA states that those involved in a trial should, when the trial finishes, be given access to the best available medicines. This is something that the FDA views as unrealistic and damaging. They say it purports to demand best-quality care for Third World trialists, but will actually just lead to fewer companies being willing to test anything in the Third World. It ties a company to providing top-quality care to people simply because they have already tried to improve the knowledge about what care is best. It rewards those patients willing to be in trials, but penalises the companies offering to do them. Forcing drug companies to deliver large amounts of care for free, in order to test their drugs, is likely to make them back away from new treatments altogether, particularly those aimed specifically at treating Third World conditions. It encourages companies to introduce their drugs with as little testing as they can get away with, which is often a dangerously small amount.

The worldwide system of drug regulation, in fact, seems set up partly to discourage medications from being properly tested. In America, there are no national ethics committees. Testing a drug requires you to persuade each hospital involved that it is reasonable to do so. Each will have different opinions, forcing you to modify your trial in different ways at different places – as though morals and experimental methods were different in Kansas from Connecticut. And in America, as in other countries, the bureaucracy of running a trial is stifling. Side effects are recorded with an eagerness that veers into insanity. If some people taking a new therapy feel nauseated, or get a headache, then that has to become part of the drug's declared side effects, something that everyone is warned about ever afterwards – even if there were *more* headaches and nausea among the people taking the placebo. If someone gets flu while on your tablet, that too can end up on the list of side effects – even if you happen to be doing the trial in the flu season and the rates of infection in your trial are lower in those on the active drug than on the placebo.

In order to protect patients from untested and experimental treatments, like thalidomide, governments around the world have set up rules. Their net effect is to make it exceedingly difficult, as well as expensive, to do any proper trials. The result is that we are not as protected as we need to be from medical ignorance.

A good example of the difficulties comes from the use of corticosteroids to treat head injuries. Corticosteroids are released by the adrenal glands in times of stress, including illness and injury. One of their actions in the body is to subdue inflammation – to keep the body's inflammatory response from becoming so overwhelming that it is self-destructive. After a traumatic brain injury the affected area swells, exactly as your ankle does following a sprain or your knee after knocking it against a table edge. The swelling is an inflammatory process, the effect of your body directing cells towards the injured brain, cells capable of fighting off infection and helping the tissue rebuild.

All of this is a generally good thing.* Room in the skull, however, is limited. A swollen brain compresses itself. For a long time doctors have worried that the inflammatory response to a bruised brain might make the injury worse. From the early 1970s they began giving corticosteroids to reduce this response, and subdue swelling within the skull. The treatment was supported by theory and, later, by animal experiments. A study from 1985 showed that cortico-

---

* The advice to put an ice-pack on a bruise or a sprain is aimed at reducing the pain and the swelling. No one has ever done the tests necessary to determine whether it slows healing as a result.

steroids reduced damage to neuronal cells in deliberately injured mice. Later, studies were done in humans, belatedly attempting to see if this effect on cells, a soft end point, translated into a meaningful effect on human recovery and survival, the ultimate hard end points.

By the end of the twentieth century, a number of randomised placebo-controlled trials had been carried out on the effects of steroids on head injuries. They were small but, taken together, they showed evidence of benefit. A systematic review of the literature in 1997 found that altogether there had been thirteen trials, covering 2,073 patients. Collating the statistics, steroids reduced the risk of death by 1.8 per cent. It sounds like a small amount, and it is, but head injuries are common. An editorial in the *British Medical Journal* in 2000 put the figure into perspective. A million people die each year from head injuries, it pointed out, and since most of those come from car crashes, and car usage is going up, the number is likely to rise. A treatment that reduced mortality by 2 per cent would save 20,000 lives a year.

The use of steroids for head injuries was not consistent. In 1995 an American study showed that they were used in two thirds of critical care centres; a British survey in 1996 found a lower rate, with only half of the UK's neurosurgical intensive care units giving the drug. Clearly doubts remained among some doctors. The combined evidence from the thirteen separate trials allowed that there might be good reason for it. Although the benefit averaged out at a 1.8 per cent reduction in deaths, that average hid a wide possible range of different impacts and it was impossible to be sufficiently confident about what the drug did. Allowing for the play of chance, the data appeared to fit either with a treatment that was almost three times as good as that average (reducing deaths by 6 per cent), or a treatment with no effect whatsoever, or even one that actually *increased* deaths (by up to about 3 per cent).

The subsequent trial proved a vast amount of work. Some people felt it should not go ahead since the data already showed evidence of likely benefit – randomising sick people to a placebo seemed unethical. Others, convinced for less good reason that the effects of steroids were likely to be bad, felt it was unethical to give anything *other* than a placebo. The trial, known as CRASH, eventually enrolled 10,008 patients at 238 different hospitals across the world. Informed consent was not possible, since the patients concerned were too sick to give it. That posed problems in getting the trial protocol accepted by the national, regional and hospital-specific ethical review boards. The organisers argued that informed consent was not relevant – all that was needed was for the treating doctor to be 'substantially uncertain' about whether steroids were likely to help the patient. If this were so, then 'the doctor in charge should take responsibility for entering such patients [into the trial], just as they would take responsibility for choosing other treatments'.

The trial looked at hard end points, both two weeks and six months after a patient's injuries. Data from a fortnight after the treatment had been given showed that steroids had a marked effect, and one that was not likely to have occurred just from chance. Death rates were increased by 3.2 per cent among the patients who received the steroids, and the large number of patients in the trial meant that there was less than a one in 10,000 chance that the result could be due to a run of bad luck in those given the drug, and good luck in those getting the placebo. Six months after their injuries, the absolute risk of death in the steroid-treated group was 3.4 per cent higher than in those who received the placebos. The CRASH trial was an overdue evaluation of an existing treatment, and one whose conclusions are now saving lives by protecting patients from a drug that was killing them.*

* A letter to the *Lancet* in 2005 showed the caution with which some in the medical profession were able to treat even the most persuasive of findings. Combining the results from CRASH with the earlier studies gave a one in a thousand chance that this apparent harm might be an illusion based on a run of luck. 'The apparent excess of deaths in these studies could be largely or wholly due to an extreme play of chance . . . the accompanying Comment [editorial] should not have described the apparent increase in mortality as indisputable.'

Properly testing a therapy is phenomenally difficult, and the difficulties are increased by the torturous regulatory processes set up to protect patients from experimental therapies. At the same time it remains frequently easy for doctors to prescribe treatments that have never been properly tested at all, just as they did with steroids in head injuries for over thirty years, killing countless tens of thousands as a result. Regulation currently makes it far easier for a doctor to give an untested drug to all of their patients – without formal consent, monitoring or ethics approvals – than to give it to only half of them as part of an organised and methodical trial. By so rigorously protecting ourselves from experimental treatments, we are opting instead to have many on the basis only of guesswork. Some of them will be killing us.

20   Aspirin and the Heart

The First World War affected the fortunes of drugs as well as nations. In Britain, dachshunds were stoned in the street because of their German heritage – and Aspirin became briefly unpopular for the same reason. There was no British patent for Bayer to lose, since the drug was first made by the Frenchman Charles Gerhardt, but there was still a trademark. The British government took the opportunity to seize it as a spoil of war and hand it out freely. When people later realised that they missed their Aspirin, they found they could now buy it without the capital letter – and from British companies, too. Across the Atlantic, supplies of Aspirin from Germany were halted by the Royal Navy. The British naval blockade did not go down well in America; at least until the German sinking of the *Lusitania*, with consequent loss of American lives, in May 1915.

Being cut off from German industry pushed America into developing her own. The phenol needed to manufacture aspirin, being a key ingredient of battlefield explosives, was hard to come by and Bayer's American subsidiary, desperate to keep production going during the war's shortages, struggled to get enough. Their solution was to employ Hugo Schweitzer, a coal tar chemist, an advocate for German interests, and a fully paid-up spy. Schweitzer contacted Thomas Edison, who was also failing to get hold of the phenol he needed to make phonograph records. Blessed with more powers of invention than most men, and partly funded by Schweitzer, Edison gave up on buying the phenol directly and set out to manufacture it himself. He used coal-tar benzene as his starting point.

Schweitzer's deal with Edison was good for almost everyone. Using money from the German secret services, Schweitzer secured a promise from Edison of 3 tons of phenol a day (roughly a quarter of his total production). The phenol would go to Bayer's US arm, who would use it for aspirin. The German government's satisfaction was in ensuring that the phenol was thereby not free to be bought up by the British for weapons.

The month after Schweitzer agreed his deal with Edison, it was destroyed. In a plot definitely unworthy of James Bond, a German spy carrying sensitive documents managed to forget his briefcase on a train. He returned to look for it, but an American secret service agent following him had picked it up. The briefcase contained details of the phenol scheme as well as lists of German sympathisers and sabotage plans. Many of the details were made public. Thomas Edison cancelled his deal with Schweitzer and sold the phenol to the American military instead, and Bayer's popularity in the country plummeted. By the end of the war their American branch had been seized and sold off.

From 1918 to 1919, when the world could have been recovering from the war, there was influenza. It infected a third of the global population. Abnormally severe, the outbreak was also peculiar in another way. Influenza, like other infections, tends to pick off the physically vulnerable – the very young and very old. This time was an exception. Of the millions who died, half were at the physical peak of their lives.

Histories of aspirin record the effectiveness of the drug in dealing with influenza. Aspirin, wrote Diarmuid Jeffreys in 2004, 'helped millions of people in their battle with the virus and undoubtedly saved many lives as a result'. Bayer today offers the same information, stating that aspirin saved 'countless lives during major flu epidemics in Europe'. As evidence, Bayer cite a German newspaper: 'As soon as you feel ill, take to your bed with a hot water bottle at your feet, drink hot camomile tea, take three Aspirin tablets a day. If you follow these rules, you'll be fit and well again in no more than a few days.'

The majority of deaths from influenza came from pneumonia, a bacterial infection of the lungs. That was not the influenza virus itself, but another germ, leaping at opportunity. Those already struck down by one illness are less capable of fighting off a second. Other sufferers died from lung damage directly caused by the virus, the air sacs where gas exchange normally occurs swelling with inflammation and filling with blood.

Against this background, it is worth remembering that aspirin makes people feel better by lowering their fevers, but that fevers are part of the body's mechanism for fighting off infection, whether viral or bacterial. The assumption that aspirin helped people with influenza is not based on any trial evidence. People felt ill and wanted to take a medicine. Doctors saw that they were feeling ill and wanted to do something to make them better. Aspirin was the mutual solution.

The estimates of the 1918 influenza pandemic suggest it infected half a billion people. It was one of the most lethal disease outbreaks in history, yet those infected were far more likely to survive than to die. It probably killed fifty to a hundred million, meaning the chance of dying if you fell ill with it was 10 to 20 per cent. Imagine for a moment a doctor seeing a vast number of patients. Suppose that they managed to treat 2,000 different people suffering from influenza, and gave aspirin to half. Altogether the doctor could expect to see between 100 and 200 deaths out of those 2,000 people. Now imagine that aspirin changed a person's chance of survival by 20 per cent – for better or for worse. From 200 deaths in each 1,000, you get a difference appearing. Those who get the aspirin might benefit – rather than 200 dying, perhaps 160 do. A difference of forty deaths between two groups of 1,000 people each.

It would be almost impossible for any doctor to personally treat and keep track of two such large groups, one treated and one untreated. Even if they had done, a failure to randomise their patients to the different options would have betrayed them. The smallest tendency to give aspirin to certain people could have meant that the two groups became profoundly different. (What if the doctor reserved the 'best' therapy for the sickest? A treatment with a genuinely good effect might appear to be lethal.) The use of aspirin for influenza was adopted without any sort of reliable trial. Doctors and patients alike were content to believe that it worked. Bayer and historians have been content to follow them.

A drug's effects, even if they are moderately large, can almost never be reliably figured out on the basis of personal experience. If that seems like a repeated point, then it is, but it was also one that history continued to show people just could not get their heads round. The assumption is that aspirin saved lives during 1918 and 1919. It might just as easily have cost them. We have no idea.

Increased global competition after the First World War prompted the German pharmaceutical industry to pay even more attention to acting as a co-ordinated conglomerate. I. G. Farben was reincarnated in a bigger and more inclusive form than ever before. It went on to subsidise the Nazis (bureaucratically as well as financially), to make eager use of slave labour, and to produce the Zyklon B that was used in the gas chambers. I. G. Farben built a plant at Auschwitz, with the intention of using the labour of those whom its gases were not killing. At the end of the war, twenty-three I. G. Farben directors were tried for war crimes. Eleven were found guilty. Fritz ter Meer, head of the plant associated with Auschwitz, defended himself on the basis that 'concentration camp victims of scientific experiments were not subject to unacceptable suffering since they were going to die anyway'.

Bayer's own account tells how, after it became a part of I.G. Farben, 'the Bayer tradition lived on . . . and the Bayer cross was used as the trademark for all of the I.G.'s pharmaceutical products.' In 1946, while still part of I.G. Farben, it began to re-establish its international presence as Bayer: 'It was clearly vital to rebuild Bayer's foreign business,' says the company. When I.G. Farben was broken up in 1951, Bayer's separate legal existence began again, based around the same four factory sites. Despite this clear perception of historical continuities much is missing from the company's summary. There is no acknowledgement on Bayer's website that the 'four year plans' designed to get the German economy ready for war were written by Farben managers for the Nazi government. It does not mention the war crime trials, nor I.G. Farben's work camp at Auschwitz and funding of Josef Mengele's experiments on imprisoned Jews. 'I feel like I am in paradise,' said an I.G. Farben employee, Dr Helmuth Vetter, speaking of the opportunities that Farben's sponsorship of Auschwitz gave him. He spent 1942 to 1944 injecting bacteria and experimental drugs into concentration camp prisoners, actions for which he was executed as a war criminal.

Eva Mozes was one of the victims of Dr Mengele's trials. Unlike the majority, she survived. 'Emotionally I have forgiven the Nazis,' she said, 'but forgiveness does not absolve any perpetrator from taking responsibility for their actions . . . I know that the ones who ran Bayer fifty years ago are all dead now. But the company today should have the courage and decency to admit their past.' On the grounds that during the war years Bayer was a part of I.G. Farben, Bayer today denies responsibility for what happened during the war. It did not technically exist. The payments and acknowledgements that it has made have simply been for 'goodwill', and not out of any obligation.

Throughout the war years, I.G. Farben continued to use the Bayer name. After his release from prison in 1956, Fritz ter Meer was appointed head of Bayer's supervisory board. The company honours his memory by administering a scholarship fund in his name and laying wreaths at his grave.

Heart disease in the 1960s was on the increase. Richard Doll and Austin Bradford Hill showed that smoking was partly to blame. Blood pressure seemed to be a factor, although no one was quite sure why so many people's seemed to be high. Fats in the blood were also implicated. A large randomised controlled trial of over 6,000 men looked at whether a range of drugs, hormones or vitamins could prevent their having second heart attacks. To their regret, the trialists found that their interventions did more harm than good. They had to step away from recommending what had seemed, when they set out, to be perfectly reasonable treatments.

This willingness to test and reject theories, rather than adopting them because of their intuitive appeal, was proof of medicine's step forwards. But with regard to heart disease, while this more humble approach was protecting people from new drugs that actually made them worse, it was not yet managing to make them better. There were only two seemingly effective drugs for heart disease.

William Withering, in late eighteenth-century Birmingham, decided that foxglove extracts were the active ingredient of a complicated local remedy. Digitalis – after the Latin name of the plant – appeared to treat the 'dropsy'. That was the contemporary name for the swelling of the feet, ankles and legs that came on when the heart beat too weakly and the circulation backed up. Digoxin, the modern chemical derived from digitalis, does the same as its herbal predecessor. In response to it, people urinate out the extra fluid that otherwise accumulates in whichever bits of their bodies are most subject to the effects of gravity.

Digitalis and digoxin were regarded as life-savers. Not until 1997 was a reliable trial set up to assess the effects of the active drug. Before then doctors based their ideas on their clinical experience and intuition, and knew that digoxin saved lives. They could see it working. The 1997 trial showed that doctors had been wrong on this point for two centuries. People who took digoxin lived no longer than those who swallowed a placebo. That was not because it was less 'natural' than chewing on a foxglove, simply because the effect of the active compound on the human body was not as miraculous as intuition suggested. Digoxin did have some benefits – the trial showed that some of the people who took it avoided some periods of hospitalisation as a result, perhaps through helping their hearts contract more forcefully – but it brought harms as well, making patients feel weak and sick and nauseated. The trained judgement of generations of physicians, when compared with the evidence from a randomised controlled trial, was found wanting.

The other useful class of drugs for heart failure were the opiates, like morphine and heroin. They made people comfortable. If someone was having angina or a heart attack, opiates took away the pain. If the patient's heart was beating weakly, and the lungs filling with fluid as a result, the drugs eased the awful feelings of suffocation and drowning. To this day, no one has done the tests to reveal whether opiates help people live or die in either situation.

Only in 1960 did it become routine for doctors to press on people's chests when their hearts stopped beating. Up until then, the accepted response was to crack open someone's ribs, stick a hand inside, grab their heart and squeeze. Death rates from heart disease have now decreased by two thirds, but improvements in resuscitation techniques account for a tiny fraction of that change. Much more of the benefit comes from the fact that you are less likely now to be a smoker.* A large proportion, however, comes from drugs. Clot busters in the hours after a heart attack are the most dramatic. Others, like the whole cocktail that wards off future heart attacks, are dull in comparison. You take them every day for years and they make you *feel* no better. They extend your life – and your ability to enjoy it in good health – all the same.

What these drugs have in common is that all of them make only *moderate* differences. None of them is like streptomycin for tuberculous meningitis, or penicillin for someone dying of overwhelming infection. None of them has effects that are big enough to understand on the basis of a doctor's personal experience. None of them, in fact, has effects big enough to be understood without the use of properly designed trials of thousands of people. Despite that, each one of them has saved vast numbers of lives. Taken together they have changed the nature of human heart disease.

The first and most important of all these drugs is aspirin.

Fever and pain are both aspects of the body's response to physical insult or derangement. The fever is aimed at making life more difficult for invading organisms, whose metabolisms are potentially more vulnerable to temperature changes than our own. Pain and malaise are also things that the body creates intentionally, part of its method for protecting itself. If you feel unwell then you do less, leaving more energy available for healing. Or perhaps you avoid using an injured part of your body, allowing it to rebuild more reliably. Celsus, a first-century AD Roman writer, described fever and pain as being two of the components of inflammation, the body's

---

* The harmful effects of smoking are roughly equivalent to the combined good ones of every medical intervention developed since the war. Those who smoke, in other words, now have the same life expectancy as if they were non-smokers without access to any health care developed in the last half-century. Getting rid of smoking provides more benefit than being able to cure people of every possible type of cancer.

overall reaction to illness or trauma. Rubor, calor, dolor and tumour were his four sonorous cardinal signs – redness, heat, pain and swelling.

To a large extent, Celsus was accurate. The body does have a generalised response to injury. We still use the term 'inflammation', although doctors are also fond of 'inflammatory cascade' (probably because it is longer). Along with the four responses that Celsus mentioned, there are others. The immune system is mobilised through various hormones. And the blood's tendency to clot is increased, a helpful response given that bodily insults are often caused by trauma that makes you bleed.

Aspirin, in a different way from thalidomide but with some of the same effects, damps down overall inflammation, interfering with the chain of biochemical changes that underlie it. Thalidomide's mechanism is not fully understood, partly because it seems to act on a variety of different biochemical reactions. Aspirin seems more precise, chiefly inhibiting an enzyme called cyclo-oxygenase which is used by the body to control the production of locally acting pro-inflammatory hormones. That is why the same drug that reduces a fever also helps relieve pain and ease swelling. And in line with its overall ability to interfere with the processes of inflammation, aspirin makes your blood less likely to clot.

In the 1960s, with the developed world increasingly frightened of heart disease, blood clots were gaining a lot of attention. Most heart disease seemed to be caused by blockages of the heart's arteries, fatty plaques that steadily developed over time. That left a puzzle as to how something that grew slowly could cause very sudden problems. The emerging conclusion was that the fatty lumps within the blood vessels really did enlarge gradually, and as they did so their surfaces became increasingly inflamed. Eventually, triggered by the inflammation, clots formed, shutting off the small spaces down which blood was flowing. If that happened in a coronary, a vessel supplying the heart with blood, you had a heart attack. A chunk of your heart muscle died. If it was a big enough portion, so did you.

The story of Lawrence Craven is a curious one, bridging the world of anecdote and quackery with the emerging one of reliable testing. Born in Iowa in 1883, Craven studied science and medicine in Minnesota, then spent the First World War as a captain in the US military. The war over, he moved to California and devoted the rest of his life to working as a family doctor. That included a lot of minor surgery. Removing large numbers of tonsils and adenoids was once thought to be an essential part of good medical care. The procedures were believed, on the basis of medical experience and medical judgement, to be extremely useful. Actual research has tended to say otherwise and rates of both operations have now plummeted. For Lawrence Craven, however, they were a big part of his working life.

Craven's first aspirin-related publication was a letter to the *Annals of Western Medicine and Surgery*. It resulted partly from his experience of performing these minor operations. He felt confident that aspirin made the blood less liable to clotting, and while this was not a new finding he did not think that it was widely enough appreciated. Craven worried about two things. First, he noted that rates of bleeding after removing someone's tonsils or adenoids were on the increase. He put this down to wider use of aspirin for pain relief. Second, he wondered whether aspirin could prevent the blood clots that caused heart attacks.

Before Craven, other doctors tried something called dicoumarol for the same purpose. Dicoumarol was discovered as the result of natural observations on cattle in 1921. Across North America, cows occasionally dropped down dead. Sometimes they were found to have small external wounds that simply never clotted. Other times they looked entirely healthy, but when vets opened them up they found massive internal bleeding. Frank Schofield, a Canadian vet, discovered that what the cows had in common was the consumption of a particular plant, sweet clover.

'Sweet clover disease' was a disorder of blood-clotting, resulting from cows eating badly cured hay that had become mouldy. Karl Link and other chemists at the University of Wisconsin managed to separate, crystallise and determine the structure of the causative molecule in the hay. Dicoumoral, as it was called, belonged to a class of naturally occurring substances called coumarins, used for their smell and their flavour in perfumes and in drinks. (Coumarins have a fragrance similar to freshly mown hay; chilled Bison grass vodka is a good example.) In 1948 Link suggested that an altered form of dicoumarol might be useful as a rat poison. In view of its being developed with the help of the Wisconsin Alumni Research Foundation, and being a coumarin, Link called the new substance warfarin.

Although clinicians had shown interest in the effects of dicoumarol on man, Link found that they were reluctant to try out the new warfarin. The fact it had been 'originally promoted to exterminate' put them off. Then, in 1951, a member of the American military attempted to kill himself using the poison. Changing his mind after five days of taking only moderate doses, he reported to a naval hospital and was looked after until the drug had worn harmlessly out of his system.

Warfarin turned out to be not only more powerful but also more clinically predictable than dicoumarol, and rapidly became the favoured medical means for reducing the blood's inclination to clot. The drug was powerful, effective and clearly dangerous. The side effects were dramatic enough to be obvious. On balance, doctors were not sure if it was useful. Aspirin, Craven suggested, was safer.

As a theory to raise, it was inspired. As something to believe in without proof, it was appalling. Aspirin was clearly a less potent drug that dicoumarol or warfarin. The side effects were rarer. Craven's assumption was that it must therefore be safe. The idea that, like dicoumarol, it offered a balance of risks, did not occur to him. To prove that aspirin reduced the blood's ability to clot, Craven swallowed aspirin until his nose began to bleed. Milder side effects, in his mind, meant ones that could be written off. Milder benefits just meant benefits.

Led on by this mental arithmetic of unthinking optimism, Craven set out to test his theory. His approach was medieval. He decided aspirin was likely to work and started handing out prescriptions. His letter to the *Annals of Western Medicine and Surgery* reported his experience of giving it daily to 400 people for two years. None of them, he said, had suffered a heart attack. Initially he thought it should be taken by all men between thirty and ninety years of age, later he dropped that to those who were forty-five to sixty-five, overweight and under-exercised.

In 1953 Craven wrote to the *Mississippi Valley Medical Journal*. By then he reported having given daily aspirin to around 1,500 people. As before, he found that not one of them had suffered a heart attack while taking the drug. His justifications for prescribing it are interesting:

The value of Aspirin (acetylsalicylic acid) in the general prophylaxis of coronary occlusion is suggested by observations accumulated during the past seven years. Concededly, the effectiveness of any type of prophylactic treatment is difficult to prove, and this applies especially to a procedure aiming merely at nonspecific prevention. Observations on healthy subjects can never be made under strictly scientific conditions, and resulting figures are only within limits suitable for statistical evaluation. Such findings may therefore merely have the value of preliminary impressions, and will be substantiated or refuted by subsequent clinical research. But as long as the field of general prophylaxis of coronary thrombosis is still outside the limits of present-day research procedures, preliminary observations may still be of practical importance provided: 1. the measure is safe in all subjects and throughout the entire extended period of medication; 2. the observations are not in opposition to the trend and results of clinical and experimental research; and 3. it is well understood that the findings were not arrived at under strictly scientific conditions.

The first sentence is fine. Leaving aside for a moment Craven's choice of recommending aspirin to everyone he knew, his observation that it reduced heart attacks was reasonable. Starting off with a suggestion of benefit, and knowing that it is only a suggestion, was a good way to begin. The second and third sentences show the mental difficulties facing an obviously intelligent and educated doctor in the years after the Second World War. Craven was aware that his methods were not scientific. That is, they relied on impressions rather than tests, and he knew that impressions were not always enough to outweigh the fantasies of the investigator. Yet not only was he unaware of methods for accurately comparing two groups of people treated with aspirin, he decided that unreliable methods were good enough to be going on with. He pointed out the flaws in his beliefs but he trusted them anyway. He had a hunch that his judgement was sound.

Craven's speculation that research techniques might improve was mistimed. The methods of the randomised, double-blind, placebo-controlled trial were already in print. The MRC streptomycin trial was published in 1948, when Craven began his 'experiments'.* Five years later he was still unaware of it. But perhaps the strangest

---

* The word too easily means trials of widely varying reliability and power to uncover truths.

conclusion that Craven reached is that aspirin 'is safe in all subjects and through the entire extended period of medication'. He had tested it on himself until his nose fountained with blood. He was proposing it as an alternative to the dicoumarol which was known to kill by causing haemorrhage. He had written about aspirin itself causing dangerous post-operative bleeding. Deciding that it was now entirely and at all times safe was exceedingly odd. We might not be totally certain of aspirin's benefits, Craven was saying, but it can't do any harm. Let's give it to everyone.

Eventually, Craven claimed to have used aspirin on 8,000 of his friends and patients. He reported that 'not a single case of detectable coronary or cerebral thrombosis occurred among patients who faithfully adhered to this regime during a period of eight years'. It is an astonishing statement. Very few treatments are so effective as to completely eliminate all cases of a disease, and we know that aspirin is not one of them.

What was the explanation for Craven's perfect results? Most likely there is a clue in the sentence's careful qualification. Craven says that there were no heart attacks (coronary thromboses) or strokes (cerebral thromboses) among those who '*faithfully adhered to this regime during a period of eight years*'. The implication is that there were both strokes and heart attacks, but that on close questioning Craven was able to satisfy himself that the patients who suffered had not been 100 per cent reliable when it came to taking their pills. This was probably true. No one is perfect at swallowing daily tablets. The advantage of not using a placebo control is that you can always come up with an explanation that handily accounts for whatever it is you want to explain away. Nine out of his 8,000 patients died, and Craven was thorough enough to make sure autopsies were performed. Some showed ruptures of the aorta, the main blood vessel emerging from the heart. Rather than being worried that these internal bleeds were due to aspirin, Craven felt vindicated that his patients had not died of heart attacks.

Craven is an excellent representation of the sort of thinking that held medicine back. He was an astute, industrious, intelligent and well-intentioned man, but those qualities could not compensate for methodological errors in the way he came to his conclusions. His suspicion of aspirin's benefits was correct, but it was a lucky guess – particularly lucky for the 8,000 people to whom he prescribed it on that basis.

The medical profession ignored Craven for all the wrong reasons. Not because of the flaws in his approach but because he was an obscure family doctor without the academic warrant to come up with interesting ideas. Cardiologists were appalled that Craven could not explain *how* aspirin stopped blood from clotting. It says something about medical thinking that this was deemed to be a valid criticism. It was entirely clear that aspirin interfered with the blood's ability to clot. The cardiologists who held the power and prestige, however, did not feel that this was important. There was no satisfying theory to explain *how* aspirin prevented blood from clotting; therefore the fact that it obviously did so was not interesting. What mattered was not demonstrable fact but missing theory.

Lawrence Craven, despite his aspirin, died from a heart attack. It was 1957 and he was seventy-four. No one responded to his thoroughly appropriate calls for more interest in aspirin and more studies of its effects. In fact, no one looked at the therapeutic potential of aspirin for heart disease for years. 'The reasons for the delay', said the *New York Times* in 1991, 'are not clear but they partly reflect the tendency of scientists to insist on understanding the biological mechanism for a treatment before studying it.' That was a polite way of saying that doctors got more pleasure from complicated theories than from simple tests. The *New York Times* also commented on why Craven's ideas were not taken up by pharmaceutical companies. Their interest was more reliably pragmatic, and much better suited to favouring proven effects over absent theories. The way the patent system was arranged, though, discouraged them from looking at aspirin. Patents get given out for drugs rather than for uses. Governments, in other words, have set up a system that rewards companies for coming up with new compounds but not for finding fresh uses for existing ones. Discovering a way of making aspirin save millions of lives was simply not something that offered strong financial incentives. Patent laws are there to reward those willing to stake their money on research. When it comes to encouraging the exploration of existing drugs, they fail.

From 1967, reports began appearing that aspirin interfered with platelets, tiny fragments within blood that cause it to clot. That helped get doctors a little more interested, but it was not decisive. The actual way in which aspirin exerted its influence was still unclear. 'Credit for influencing physicians to prescribe aspirin for heart problems', says Gabriel Khan, a Canadian cardiologist, in his 2005 *Encyclopedia of Heart Diseases*, 'must be given to John Vane.' Dr Khan's justification is that it was John Vane who finally described the molecular mechanism by which aspirin operated.

Lovely as it was, in terms of showing how it was that aspirin affected platelets and, through them, blood clots and then cardiologists, Vane's work was not what prodded physicians into motion. John O'Brien did more. A haematologist (blood specialist) working in Portsmouth, England, he was unaware of Craven but also published a paper (this time in 1963) showing that aspirin prevents blood clots. O'Brien's innovation was to show, by using measurements of platelet stickiness, that fairly routine doses of aspirin had clear effects. O'Brien was deliberately trying to find drugs that inhibited blood clots. Before reading about aspirin, he tried a range of other drugs. Some of them stopped clots, but only at doses that were likely to kill people. Once he felt confident about aspirin, O'Brien followed his first paper up with a *Lancet* article in 1968. There he suggested a trial of the drug for preventing heart attacks. By then others were thinking along the same lines.

Sometime in 1968, O'Brien met up with Peter Elwood, a doctor whose interest in epidemiology had led to him to take up a post with Archie Cochrane in Wales. O'Brien had already tried to persuade the MRC to pay for a trial of aspirin in heart disease, but his calculations of the number of people required made the prospect too expensive. The effects of aspirin were likely to be moderate, reasoned O'Brien, and so large numbers of patients needed to be enrolled into any trial that was going to be able to distinguish the effects of aspirin from the shifting fortunes of chance. Elwood came up with an improvement. What was needed, he realised, was not so much a large number of people as a large number of actual heart attacks. A trial recruiting only those at high risk of heart attacks would need fewer people. And since one heart attack often predicted another, you had a straightforward way of identifying a large group of people who were definitely at risk.

This time the Medical Research Council was persuaded. A randomised, double-blind, placebo-controlled trial was set up and, from 1970, began enrolling patients. Archie Cochrane, still convinced that cardiologists deserved constructive mockery, taunted them that their expensive coronary care units might be made redundant by something as old and cheap as aspirin.

John Crofton had found his involvement in the MRC streptomycin investigations less than inspiring – trials, he concluded, were important but 'not intellectually challenging'. Elwood was the other way around. Having been bored as a junior doctor, he found the world of trials altogether different. 'I found it so intellectually intoxicating I used to walk home reading a textbook and often I would get so entranced I'd walk into a lamp-post.' (Jeffreys, 2004)

On a Saturday in 1972, Elwood was in his office. The phone rang. It was a call from an American pharmacologist named Herschel Jick, working in Boston. Jick was involved in a study looking at what drugs patients were taking during the few days before coming into hospital. It was a trawl to see if they could pick up associations, good or bad – and, like all trawls, it had a high likelihood of fishing out something meaningless. Jick's trawl involved forty different diseases and around sixty different drugs. Even if every one of those drugs was an identical placebo, that meant you could expect to find some relationships that looked meaningful when they weren't.

However, the association that Jick's team discovered did not sound at all meaningless to Elwood. Heart attack patients were taking a third less aspirin than others. If Jick's finding was not chance, it meant that people on aspirin were coming into hospital with heart attacks much less than expected. That implied one of two explanations. Either aspirin was preventing heart attacks, or it was making them so much worse that patients never made it to the hospital alive.

The use of speculative studies that go looking for associations is in turning up hypotheses. You find a link between admission rates and aspirin and you theorise to yourself that it is not just there by chance. Then you set up an interventional study to figure out whether it really is cause and effect. You give some people aspirin and see what happens. You carry out a study, in other words, exactly like the one that Elwood and O'Brien had laboriously set up. Jick's team wanted Elwood to dissolve their trial, to end it prematurely just in case they were killing people with aspirin. 'Look,' they said, 'we have to know if aspirin is beneficial or harmful.'

When it comes to designing a trial, or understanding a treatment, certain outcomes matter more than others. The ones that ultimately count are called 'hard' outcomes. Others, often used because they are easier to count and collect, act as proxies. They are 'soft' outcomes. For aspirin and heart attacks, Elwood's team were using the hardest outcome of all – death. That was what they felt really mattered; did the drug help people survive?

They could have chosen softer outcomes. Not everyone who has a heart attack dies from it, for example. If you count heart attacks instead of deaths then your trial is quicker and easier and cheaper. There are simply more heart attacks than deaths. Elwood and O'Brien were concerned that, since aspirin was a pain killer, it might stop people from noticing a small heart attack. (Even without drugs, some heart attacks are curiously painless.) In other words, they felt that the number of observed heart attacks would be a poor proxy for figuring out the actual effects of aspirin. The soft outcome was not reliable enough. The drawback of their trial's high quality was that it needed to recruit large numbers of people, enough that a sufficient number would die. A difference in deaths between two groups – or enough observed deaths to show no difference at all – was needed to determine what aspirin actually did.

Elwood pointed out to Jick that the MRC trial of aspirin had so far recorded only seventeen deaths. If aspirin were a miracle drug, with a massive effect, those seventeen might be enough to reveal the truth about it – if all seventeen had been taking the placebo, say, or if all of them had been on the real drug. Aspirin was not new, though, and despite Craven's suggestion that it stopped every single heart attack and stroke, no one believed that its effects could possibly be that overwhelming. So seventeen deaths were too few to make the trial meaningful. What the American team were asking did not really make sense. Stopping a trial early means you get results sooner, but it also increases your chances of them being useless or misleading. In order to go along with the American request, Elwood's and O'Brien's trial needed to remove the double-blinding that kept secret who was on aspirin and who on placebo. That meant compromising their trial.

Oddly, and after some debate, Elwood and Cochrane agreed with the American request. Eleven of the patients who had died turned out to be taking placebos, six aspirin. As predicted, it was meaningless. Aspirin neither killed everyone nor saved everyone.

Those numbers were too small and similar to be taken as saying anything else.

Reassured that their patients were not all dropping dead as the result of their aspirin, Elwood and his colleagues correctly concluded that their trial efforts needed to be started up again. They did so, reporting in 1974 on their subsequent recruitment of 1,239 men with recent heart attacks. Giving half of them aspirin and half a placebo, they got results that were suggestive of the drug's helping to keep people alive. But they were not conclusive.

There is no absolute guarantee that *any* result is not the work of chance. The more unlikely it is, though, the more confident you can be. The chance that Elwood's trial was due to luck, rather than an effect from aspirin, was more than one in twenty, and therefore over the conventional cut-off for statistical significance.

The result of the aspirin trial persuaded some doctors to start prescribing it for those at risk of a heart attack. More usefully, it encouraged others to make their own attempts at similar trials. The larger the number of people studied, the more confidence you could have in the results. What was continuing to be clear was that aspirin was not a magic cure; the sort of impact that Craven reported simply did not exist. And the difficulty of proving moderate effects, ones that were often not apparent for some time after someone began swallowing a pill, were substantial.

The Medical Research Council, with Elwood and Cochrane, tried again. This time they recruited around 2,000 people to take either aspirin or a placebo. Again, the results were positive but inconclusive. 'Well, gentlemen,' said Richard Doll to the disappointed team, 'the evidence may not be certain, but it is more convincing than that for most of the other drugs in the *British Pharmacopoeia*.'

Kerr White, a friend and colleague of Cochrane's, recalled the two of them attending a conference in 1976 in New Zealand. Nervous of scaring his audience, a 'staid group of white-coated clinicians', White suggested to them that only 15 to 20 per cent of what doctors did for their patients was actually proven to work. 'In mid-sentence Archie suddenly called out: "Kerr, you're a damned liar, you know perfectly well that it isn't more than 10%!"' Both men were drawing their figures from a study of family doctors across Britain which had shown that only 9 per cent of all prescriptions written were for drugs whose effectiveness was properly established. That, after all the years of medical advances, was the extent to which doctors knew what they were doing.

Neither the two Medical Research Council trials nor another four done across the world showed a conclusive answer for aspirin. The last one reported in 1980, and after it appeared Cochrane and Elwood attempted to combine the results from all six. Finally, they thought, they had something persuasive. Altogether almost 11,000 people had been treated with aspirin as part of one of these randomised, double-blind, placebo-controlled trials. Put together, the numbers became convincing. If you started taking aspirin after having a heart attack, your chance of dying went down by around a quarter. Cochrane and Elwood calculated the odds of a genuinely useless pill giving such good results by chance. This time they came out at less than one in 10,000.

Aspirin decreased a patient's chance of dying by a quarter in the year after their heart attack. A big effect, but too small to be reliably apparent on the basis of a doctor's clinical experience. Too small even to show up in trials involving 2,000-odd patients.

The benefits of aspirin are, in some ways, certain. If you give the pill to a large number of people, you save lives. It does a population good. On any given occasion, for any given patient, however, it can be useless. Swallow an aspirin after your heart attack, and there is a chance – a risk – that it will save your life. There is also a chance it will do nothing, and a chance it will make you bleed. Some of those bleeds go on to kill.

Before the introduction of aspirin, 88 per cent of people survived their heart attacks. By helping to prevent blood clots in coronary arteries, aspirin improved that number. Without aspirin the chances of dying were 12 per cent. Cut that by a quarter, and it went down to 9 per cent. In other words, if you give people a pill that improves their survival by a quarter, the effects you see depend very much on how likely they were to die in the beginning. Given that most people survive heart attacks, the impact of aspirin can seem minor. Rather than 88 per cent of people surviving a heart attack, 91 per cent do.

Aspirin drops your risk of dying by a quarter, your *relative risk*. Your overall chance of dying, however, goes from 12 per cent to 9 per cent – your *absolute risk* reduces by 3 per cent. Craven may have had some good ideas, but his results were not even close to being right. The only way he could have got the numbers he did was by introducing bias. That is not to say he *consciously* manipulated anything, only that it takes something as strict and careful as a randomised, double-blind, placebo-controlled trial for even the most humane and sincere people to avoid doing so. That 3 per cent is not enough for any doctor – even a cardiologist – to dependably notice in day-to-day clinical experience. Yet it matters. Heart attacks are common. Aspirin, properly used, saves 100,000 lives worldwide, every year: about 7,000 people per year in Britain, almost 30,000 a year in America.

21 Large Trials and Grand Designs

By 1980 the need to investigate medicines reliably had become increasingly apparent. Those attracted to the effort were faced with two problems. One they knew about before they began: doctors were ignorant about the effects of most treatments. The other came as a surprise. Even when real evidence was placed in front of them, doctors sometimes took no notice of it. Habit was strong and clever explanations appealed more to clinicians than straightforward and partly statistical proofs. Researchers did not just need to change medical minds, they needed to win hearts.

It is difficult to shift fixed opinion. Two early randomised, double-blind, placebo-controlled trials were performed on homeopathy in the nineteenth century, the first in 1835, the second from 1879 to 1880. Both showed homeopathic medication did nothing different from an identically presented placebo. The *British Medical Journal* even drew doctors' attention to the second of the two trials, lauding the homeopaths for their involvement, saying it was 'highly creditable to those who ventured on an experiment involving so much peril to a favourite theory'. Neither trial, though, was understood. Failing to be convinced by either the results or the methods, believers in homeopathy went on prescribing remedies proven to be useless. Traditional doctors marched back to treatments that were even worse. The power and clarity of methodical testing were ignored.

So it seemed that doctors were merely repeating history when they took remarkably little notice of the combined aspirin trials. They did not trust them; statistical techniques were something they did not understand and did not like. The drug had been proven useful, but doctors were not using it.

'Archie was immensely gratified', said Elwood, 'when, around this time, Richard Peto took up the matter of aspirin and presented a considerably elegant overview.' What Peto, a statistician with medical interests, did was to take the data from the six trials of aspirin in heart disease, and put them together in a more statistically adept – and therefore more persuasive – manner. This helped, but only a little. The medical profession remained largely impervious.

Here is Dr Khan, writing in his *Encyclopedia of Heart Diseases* about the further development of aspirin as a treatment. 'The timely 1983 study by Lewis *et al.* in the United States heralded a new era, and aspirin became widely known as a life-saving drug.' He explains that the trial demonstrated tremendous benefit, dropping rates of heart attacks by a half in those with angina. (Angina is the shortened form of 'angina pectoris', the old and still current description of the pain people feel when their hearts are starved of blood; in the original Latin, it means a throttling pain about the chest: a cramp of the heart. Sometimes people say they feel as if they are about to die – as, indeed, some of them are.

The 1983 study that Khan refers to came after Richard Peto's much more reliable synthesis of the aspirin trials showing that the drug extended lives. Peto's overview involved very many more patients and it showed a change in a more important outcome – heart attacks matter; staying alive matters more. Yet cardiologists were unpersuaded by Peto, just as they were by Elwood and Cochrane before them. Khan is mistaken, too, in suggesting they paid much attention to Lewis's study of 1983. Cardiologists thought very little of aspirin, and following their eminent lead the family doctors who might have prescribed aspirin were also unconvinced.

There is something charming about Khan's retrospective optimism. He shows a wishful belief that cardiologists quickly understood the importance and relevance of the high-quality evidence that, for the first time, was being placed in front of them. He suggests that after ignoring the early conclusive evidence, they were open-minded enough to pay attention to the subsequent data. It is an amiable belief, but it is also wrong.

Cardiologists continued to be enchanted with their favourite theories, and indifferent to demonstrable facts. Aspirin was not new enough or powerful enough to appeal. They preferred warfarin, dicoumarol and other anticoagulants, drugs that you could really *see* working because they caused a lot of patients to bleed dramatically. Many died from their blood loss, which hammered home to the cardiologists the impression that their drugs were potent. And cardiologists, like all doctors, had a proud history of bleeding people to death while convincing them that it was for their own good. (Anticoagulants for heart attacks were later investigated with a large, randomised, double-blind, placebo-controlled trial. It found them to be useless.)

Backing up the cardiologists was the American Food and Drug Administration. At the tail end of 1980, the FDA refused permission for a drug company, Sterling, to start recommending aspirin on the basis of the new trial data. The company wanted to say that aspirin, in the wake of Peto's overview, 'has been shown to be effective in reducing the risk of death or re-infarction of patients who have suffered a myocardial infarction', meaning a heart attack. The FDA, as unable to understand the evidence as most cardiologists, forbade Sterling from doing so. The importance of this was that it affected advertising. Aspirin was registered as a drug to treat fevers and pain. Without the FDA's approval, companies were not allowed to market it for treating heart disease. Sterling was already taking a risk in trying to invest in aspirin, since the patent for it was long expired. Now the FDA was forbidding it from even advertising in order to try to familiarise doctors with the drug's proven benefits. Doctors could still prescribe it for heart attack victims if they wished – they were under no compulsion to pay any attention to what the FDA thought – but few of them thought that it was of any use in such situations.

In 1983, Sterling had another go. This time it got as far as persuading the FDA to formally listen to the case. Sterling flew over Peto and Elwood to present their data. The committee listened happily to the speaker who came first, a man who explained the theories behind why aspirin should work to prevent heart attacks.

Diarmuid Jeffreys' *Aspirin*, a history of the drug, gives a wonderful account of the collision that followed, when the British doctors stepped up to speak. The committee distrusted the data from Elwood's two MRC trials. And, more importantly, they were unconvinced by Richard Peto's claim that the results from different trials could be usefully combined to give a robust conclusion.

> Dressed in his customary brown corduroy jacket, with no tie and with longish blond hair falling over his collar, Peto cut an unusual figure in a room full of conservatively suited executives. He clearly anticipated that his ideas were going to be challenged and he was in no mood to be patronized by an American panel that he suspected held unflattering views of British science . . . His *ad hoc* style was more informal than the panel members were used to and his ironic tone seemed to suggest that if the Americans couldn't see what he was on about, it was their failing not his.

Elwood recalled that the meeting collapsed. Peto, upset, was reduced to calling people fools and idiots. Sterling was denied permission to market aspirin to heart attack victims.

Over a year later, in December 1984, the FDA heard Sterling's case again. This time Peto dressed both himself and his talk up with all the paraphernalia and style that the committee expected. Rather than scribbling out explanations as he went, he had slides. Rather than corduroy, he wore a suit.

> You will hear some doctor saying, well, if it doesn't show up in a trial with a couple of hundred patients then it can't be worth bothering with. This is not medical wisdom but statistical unwisdom.

Interventions that exert moderate effects on common diseases, Peto explained, can save a lot of people's lives.

> Some of these people will be old, some will be horrible people who would be better dead anyway, but a fair number of these are going to be in middle age with a reasonable chance of enjoying life. So this kind of thing is worth doing.

This time the committee was convinced. The FDA approved labelling aspirin as a life-saving treatment for those with heart disease. A year later the US Health Secretary was explaining the drug's benefits to the press.

Jeffreys' account is a vivid one, but it makes no mention of the cost of the delay. In between the FDA's rejecting Sterling's first presentation and accepting the second, heart disease carried on its normal business of killing. In America alone, 20,000 people died that year whom aspirin would have kept alive. The FDA's jurisdiction only applies to America, but its influence is worldwide. The impact of the FDA's delay was huge. So was the delay of governments worldwide in advertising aspirin's benefits. Why was there a year's gap between FDA approval and the US Health Secretary holding up a packet of aspirin at a press conference? Even when science provided firm answers, bureaucrats were slow to respond.

Aspirin was gradually taken up, in the wake of academic papers and conference presentations, advertisements and press conferences. Dr Khan's encyclopedia suggests that by 1983, cardiologists had enthusiastically adopted it as a treatment for heart disease. The British Heart Foundation looked, in 1987, to see if that was true. They counted how often coronary care units – the pinnacle of cardiological practice – gave aspirin to their patients. Of those for whom it was potentially life-saving, it was being given to one in ten.

The original meaning of the term 'antibiotic' was not a substance that helped snuff out an infecting bug, but something that one organism's physiology manufactured in order to wage war with another. Some of these bugs, having evolved to attack us, produce molecules tailored by natural selection to do so. And in the same way that all beneficial drugs have the capacity to harm, some harmful ones are also able to help.

The streptococcus that causes puerperal fever no longer preys so much upon mothers. There are occasional cases, but the last epidemic outbreak was in 1965 in Boston, Massachusetts. The reason for the decline is not understood, but may represent the bacteria's having evolved to focus on other things than causing disease, or at least this disease. Nevertheless, the streptococcus is still around, and still retains much of its basic molecular equipment. One of the ways in which it was deadly was through its production of a drug acting on human blood. It is a molecule that stops clots from forming, or breaks them up if they are already there. From the point of view of the streptococcus, the drug helps it avoid being walled off by a host's defences, entombed within a blood clot.

From the 1950s, doctors were experimenting with a drug made

out of the molecule. It was called streptokinase and it dissolved blood clots regardless of whether bacteria were present. During the following decades, trials were undertaken to see if it could usefully attack the clots that form in coronary arteries. By the time the FDA approved the change in labelling for aspirin, streptokinase had been generally rejected. It was clearly dangerous – causing far more bleeding even than the anticoagulant drugs – and the trials of it were disappointing. True, they were all too small to actually give a reliable answer, but the cardiologists were not going to have their decision-making slowed down by such quibbles. They had carried out a few trials and now they were ready to move on to trying something else.

Combining the results of lots of small trials – putting similar experiments together to increase the validity of their conclusions – was, however, starting to become popular. Richard Peto was involved in an overview combining the data from thirty-three separate trials of streptokinase. Individually, each was so small as to be meaningless. Taken together, they showed something surprising: streptokinase was dangerous, but it worked. It caused more fatal bleeding than aspirin, but it also stopped more fatal heart attacks. On balance, it did good and saved lives. Together with two colleagues, the cardiologist Salim Yusuf and the trials specialist Rory Collins, Richard Peto published this analysis in a specialist cardiology journal. Most cardiologists who read their paper did not believe it.

Faced with a group of specialists who understood so little about the nature of medical knowledge, the researchers came up with another strategy. They had uncovered the truth about aspirin and streptokinase, and most cardiologists had ignored them. Now they looked for ways to get the cardiologists to do better. Doctors could clearly not be relied on to understand scientific method; attention had to be paid to educating them.

A large trial was therefore designed with a dual purpose. It was an attempt to alert cardiologists to the nature of reality, but also designed to uncover a bit of new knowledge along the way. What happened, for example, if you gave streptokinase *and* aspirin? Given that streptokinase carried such a risk of terrific blood loss, was there a way of figuring out exactly those people it was either likely to kill or to save, so as to more profitably choose whom to give it to?

The new trial was so large that, rather than being listed under the names of those organising it, it had its own name. There were too many people involved (and perhaps too many medical egos) to name it any other way. ISIS-2 was actually the second in a series. The first International Study of Infarct Survival had looked at drugs called beta blockers, and their ability to help people live through their heart attacks. This second one now took 17,000 heart attack patients and divided them into four groups. One group got aspirin, another streptokinase, a third both; the fourth group got nothing at all. Given the fact that both aspirin and streptokinase were already proven to save lives, a control group that got neither was an ethically curious decision.

The trial published its results in 1988. Of the patients who got nothing at all, 87 per cent survived to the end of the month after their heart attack. Aspirin improved things, and so did streptokinase. In fact, the two drugs worked out pretty much the same, improving people's chances by similar amounts (just over a 2 per cent absolute increase in survival rates for each) despite that fact that one had dramatic results – both good and bad – while the other was milder. Given together, they provided the best of all outcomes. Among that group, 92 per cent survived at the end of the month. Taken together, these two drugs reduced someone's chance of dying from a heart attack, their relative risk, by about 40 per cent.

This time, the trial was so big and so conclusive that people took notice. The British Heart Foundation had found that 10 per cent of heart attack patients were being given aspirin the year before ISIS-2 came out. The year after it was published, in 1989, they repeated their survey. This time the figure was 90 per cent.

The research unit that Richard Peto helped to set up continues to operate, to undertake large trials and report on their effects. They estimate that aspirin prevents around 4,000 deaths a year in Britain alone. If everyone who was meant to be on it actually was, and all those people took their tablets, that number would be 7,000. Medicine's main benefits for human health are in these accretions of moderate effects.

'What needs to be overcome', said William Silverman, an American paediatrician energised by the battle to do his patients more good than harm, 'is a naïve "all-*and*-none concept".' A patient within a double-blind, randomised controlled trial is taking a risk. One of the treatments is likely to be better than another, and patients have no control over which one they get. In the case of ISIS-2, some of the harm could have been avoided by getting rid of the placebo arm – in other words, if cardiologists had been a touch more modest and an ounce more numerate, an estimated seventeen deaths would have been avoided among the trial patients alone. (To a significant extent, cardiology is now a speciality that has learnt its lesson. That is to say, many treatments within cardiology are now based on good evidence. Many others are not.)

What is needed is a culture, regulatory and intellectual, where every attempt is made to ensure new medical interventions are used solely in randomised trials. Only when their effects have been determined should they become available for use outside a trial setting. Until then there is a moral obligation on doctors to use unknown drugs and treatments only in such a way as to come to an understanding of them, and a moral obligation on patients to demand treatments that are either supported by sound evidence, or only given as part of a trial which will uncover some.

No regulatory system can encourage all innovation and stifle all errors. No amount of trials can make sure that all medical decisions are based on the firmest conceivable evidence. That is no reason not to keep trying.

22   The Battle for Hearts and Minds

Around a quarter of a century ago doctors began using a new type of drug to treat their patients.

Although some of those with heart disease are killed by clots in their coronary arteries, others die in different ways. The electrical co-ordination of the heart, particularly in past sufferers of heart attacks, can go wrong. Rather than beating, the heart just quivers. This is precisely the condition for which people are given electric shocks. The paddles on their chest deliver a charge that can reset the heart's conducting system. As a medical approach, it has more than a little in common with switching a computer off and on again. Sometime it works, sometimes not.

On the reasonable grounds that prevention was better than cure, cardiologists tried to think of ways of protecting the heart from these sorts of problems. They noticed that there were certain patterns of electrical activity that predicted future disaster. Everyone's heart skips out of its normal rhythm, at least a few times each day. It throws in extra beats and misses the odd one or two as well. After a heart attack, though, people with lots of extra beats seemed to be at higher risk of dropping down dead from a sudden and total electrical failure of cardiac co-ordination.

A class of drugs were developed − antiarrhythmics − that prevented these extra beats. This was where doctors let themselves down. They reasoned that if you suppressed the extra beats, people would live longer. As a theory it was perfectly respectable, but theories are hypotheses that you test. Whereas cardiologists had once been suspicious of aspirin because of their inability to explain the mechanism by which it thinned the blood, with antiarrhythmics they seemed content to behave in a very different way. Perhaps because these drugs were newer, and linked in their minds with all the allure of modern technology, they were far more confident about them. Whatever the reasons, they aware of the gap in their knowledge but believed it did not matter. Why go to the trouble of testing drugs that were so obviously going to work? Why delay the introduction of potentially life-saving medication?

This line of thought was set out explicitly by a doctor called Bernard Lown, speaking at the 1978 convention of the American College of Cardiology. Four hundred thousand people a year were dying suddenly when their hearts stopped, said Lown. The way to help save them was to stop the extra heartbeats that came before their deaths. He admitted that there was no direct proof that preventing the beats prevented the deaths, but when people were dying at such a rate, what purpose could be served by waiting to confirm the theory? 'In medicine,' he explained, 'great rewards have flowed from partial answers and usually have preceded complete solutions. This is the case with sudden cardiac death.'

A few doctors disagreed, and said they thought this partial knowledge was not enough. They suggested that experiments needed to be done in order to show that the drugs suppressing the extra heartbeats were actually life-saving. They got very little attention. 'In American medicine,' said Thomas Moore, who wrote a book about the whole shambolic episode, 'words of caution rarely slow the rush to treatment.' The thought was in tune with Oliver Wendell Holmes's ideas about the American longing for heroic cures, but allocating blame to Americans in particular seems unreasonable. The drugs also began to be used eagerly in Europe and elsewhere. The Soviet Union developed a novel one of their own.

The idea that suppressing extra beats was life-saving took hold in the 1970s. At the end of the decade, in 1979, American doctors were writing out 12 million prescriptions a year for these drugs, trying to keep the hearts of their nation beating along in an orderly fashion. By 1981, an editorial in the *New England Journal of Medicine* praised their utility. One such drug was described as 'an important addition to the current antiarrhythmic armamentarium'. If that last word sounds pre-modern, almost medieval, than so was the untested thought behind it.

For the best part of a hundred years, America had already possessed regulation claiming to make sure drugs were safe and effective before they were used. Each time a drug disaster showed the regulation to be a mockery, it was improved a little bit. Never enough, but a little. In the 1970s and 1980s the requirement to prove effectiveness still did not specify how 'effectiveness' should be measured. In this case the drugs were effective in the eyes of the cardiologists; that was enough for the FDA, and enough for the cardiologists themselves. Today there is still no absolute requirement for proving hard end points like mortality. A soft proxy, in this case the suppression of extra beats, is often still acceptable.

To begin with, the main avenue for prescribing these drugs was through 'compassionate use exemptions' allowing the use of experimental drugs on people too sick to wait for tests to be completed. The whole idea of the exemptions is based on the presumption that they are likely, once the testing has been finished off, to actually work. This is itself based on the belief that new drugs are more likely to help than harm. Compassionate use allows the drugs to be prescribed outside a trial. It often supplies doctors with their earliest experiences of a treatment. Thus the medical profession frequently forms its views on the basis of anecdotes, of observations without any of the trappings even of second-rate methodology. The drugs, thought the doctors, worked well. The extra heartbeats were effectively suppressed. Some of the patients died, but then they were people with damaged hearts. Doubtless some were always going to die. The cardiologists reckoned that there would have been more deaths if not for their new drugs.

The first attempt to test any of these drugs came with one called flecainide in 1983. Flecainide interferes with the way heart cells use sodium ions to control their contractions, altering the overall way in which the heart beats.

As so often, when doctors are persuaded to trial something, the aim was not to see if their theories were correct. They were certain about that. Their aim was to persuade *other* doctors, whose intuitions were different. This first study was in fifty-five patients. That turned out, as could have been easily predicted, to be too small a number to determine the drug's actual effects. The next study, this time of 630 people and of a similar drug called mexiletine, also ended up being too small to give an answer. That was partly because, when more people started dying in the treatment group than the placebo one, the study was brought to an early halt. It was not heading towards proving the benefit that the doctors knew was there, so there was no point in carrying on with it. The drug, noted the trial summary, appeared to be good at controlling abnormal heartbeats. That was enough for now.

At a cardiology meeting in Bermuda in the same year, 1983, paid for by the makers of flecainide, opinions about the drug were still positive. The doctors remained aware of the trial data they were missing, and remained happy that these were not essential. 'We do not need to hold up marketing of the drug until we have all of this information,' said one. Although entering any of their patients into a trial required an intimidating amount of paperwork, and a formal ritual of informed consent, simply giving it to them without any reliable trials needed none.

By 1984, the issue was still undecided. Some experts thought the drugs worked, a few did not. In the absence of any reliable trials, there was nothing better to go on than opinion. The FDA approved flecainide on the basis that the cardiologists believed in it. They noted that a minority of doctors were worried that flecainide was dangerous. Therefore, suggested the FDA, its use 'should be reserved for patients in whom, in the opinion of the physician, the benefits of treatment outweigh the risks'. Given that the physicians had nothing to base that decision on besides their own optimism, what happened next was not a surprise. Prescriptions of the drugs kept rising.

At the heart of the FDA's thinking, and it was betrayed in their words, was the old idea that benefits are certain but harms are not. And there was no conception that opinions, regardless of a doctor's personal attributes, are no way to assess risks.

Thomas Moore's history of these antiarrhythmics, *Deadly Medicine*, notes another problem. The amount of money that companies spent advertising their drugs was greater than their expenditure on research. And their research cost billions of dollars a year. In the views of the doctors, those advertising budgets did not matter. Only a tiny minority of doctors believed their own views were ever swayed by something so crude a thing as advertising. They were sure their decisions were based on an ability to weigh up rationally what was best for their patients. Good evidence, however, said that doctors were mistaken. In one study, when they were shown identical drugs advertised in different ways, half of all doctors thought that one of them was very much better than the other. Time and again research showed that doctors were influenced by advertising; this remained something that the doctors themselves could not quite believe.

So not only were doctors incapable of asking for hard evidence, they were also unaware of the degree to which their opinions were formed for them by drug company marketing. Regulatory bodies were not making sure that drugs were reliably and accurately tested, and doctors were not noticing. Given the failure of the government and the medical profession to do any better, it seems slightly unreasonable to blame the drug companies for taking advantage of the situation.

This held proper research back for years. Eventually though, starting in 1987, a large-scale, double-blind, randomised controlled trial of these heart drugs began. As with the earlier, smaller trials the goal was not to test the drugs but to convince the unbelievers and persuade them to prescribe more. Those involved in the trial already knew that the drugs worked. They even pushed for the study – a $40 million affair, spread over a hundred hospitals – to be designed in such a way as to look *only* for evidence of benefits. Anything else, they thought, was a waste of time and money. The drug companies seemed genuinely pleased. They were not cynically selling a product that they secretly knew to be poisonous. They simply shared the untested optimism of the majority of cardiologists. Given the fearsome restrictions in place since thalidomide, the trial was difficult and expensive and laborious – but a few enthusiasts got it running all the same.

The trial almost failed. It required doctors to enter their patients into a study without knowing whether they would get a placebo or one of the active drugs. There were three drugs in the trial, flecainide, encainide and moricizine, all from the class that suppressed extra heartbeats. In the views of many working doctors, the trial was unethical: the drugs were clearly good. Many cardiologists refused to let their patients near it. A shortage of willing participants almost made the whole thing impossible. Of those suitable for the trial, two thirds were ruled out because their doctors advised them that the drugs definitely worked, and that to end up on a placebo might kill them.

The trial was due to run for five years but, in April 1989, after only two, it was stopped early. All the drugs successfully stopped the extra heartbeats. They also stopped the heart. Two of the three drugs – encainide and flecainide – were shown to be killing people. The idea that the beats caused people to die turned out, on testing, to be wrong.

Details of the trial results were revealed to those involved on a Monday morning, but not immediately made public. That same Friday one of the lead investigators was attacked at a meeting about the trial. 'You are immoral!' cried out one of the cardiologists in the audience. They were not angry about the trial results; they did not yet know about them. They were angry about the trial. The drugs so plainly worked, the cardiologist was arguing, that testing them against a placebo was murderous and unethical.

Together, the two drugs that the trial showed to be harmful are thought to have actively killed around 50,000 people in America alone. A tiny number compared to those whose lives were ended by leeches, by bleeding and by the treatments that doctors practised through most of history, but the result of the same mode of thinking, the same mental habit of doctors believing their own intuitions.

As the findings of the trial were publicised, many doctors ignored them. They continued to believe their own opinions, their anecdotal experience that the drugs helped people. All of them had given the drugs to some people who then did well. They objected that if they stopped the drugs, some of their patients would die. 'Yes,' replied the aghast FDA, 'but fewer.'

Other doctors simply switched their patients to different drugs in the same class, a choice that competing pharmaceutical companies were happy to encourage. These other drugs had no proven harms since they had undergone none of the rigorous tests that might have uncovered them. They too supposedly provided benefits by suppressing extra heartbeats. Many doctors continued to believe that they simply had to work. After all, it made sense. A second trial was undertaken of the agent that was not shown to kill in the first, moricizine. That second trial was also stopped early when an excess of people on moricizine died.

The greatest failure was not that doctors were shown to be killing so many of their patients. It was that learning that they were doing so did so very little to shift their beliefs. Some of the other new drugs in the same class were subsequently also proven to kill. The fashion for using them slipped, but did not disappear. 'How much evidence was enough to persuade doctors to abandon a theory', asked Moore, 'that had been accepted without proof in the first place?' Some doctors just thought these drugs *should* work. On that basis they were willing to carry on using them.

'Doctors', notes Moore at the end of his book, 'are still free to exercise their medical judgment and may prescribe [these drugs] for patients with premature beats.'

23   The Risks of Opinion

There are too many possibilities in the world to test them all. We pick the ones that seem most likely on the basis of our theories or our previous experience. Science, when it comes to generating testable hypotheses, is an art.

Our pre-judgement might be that a new molecular drug will treat a disease, or that a traditional herb will save a life. Those are both decent reasons for setting out to see if they will, particularly if similar molecules or herbs have turned out to be helpful in the past. Pre-judgements are the best possible reasons for doing tests; they are the worst possible replacements for them. And tests need to be designed so that they can prove us wrong, no matter how strongly we believe that they won't.

There is a widespread prejudice in favour of traditional treatments. People find it difficult to believe that therapies used for hundreds or thousands of years should actually be useless. Another prejudice is contradictory – as well as liking to believe that age-old treatments must have something to them, we are also fond of favouring whatever seems most modern.

Doctors are just as subject to these two prejudices as any other people. And when it comes to testing new therapies, it is the second of the two that really worries them. From the days when control groups began to become routine in medical tests, doctors have convulsed themselves with anxiety over the unfairness. Their presumption that the new treatment will be better than the old is strong. They worry that patients in a control group are being unethically treated, denied the best opportunity of a cure or comfort.

If this is generally true, as it was in ISIS-2, then there is a real problem with clinical trials. They might be good for society, good for the majority of human beings, but they will be operating at the expense of the people within them, the people who get a placebo or the oldest of the possible treatment options.

Since proper trials began, doctors and interested observers have fretted over the extent to which they asked participants to make unreasonable sacrifices. If you could be confident that all the options being tried out were equally likely to succeed, then you could enter the trial with a glad heart. From a selfish perspective, if new treatments are likely to be better than old then patients should avoid trials at all costs. They should instead try to get hold of whatever doctors think most likely to work. And doctors should encourage them to do this. You trust that a doctor will act in *your* best interests, not those of society at large.

All of these anxieties have been particularly disturbing to doctors who look after children with cancer. Forty years ago, about three in ten children with the disease were cured. Today, that has risen to more than seven in ten. Over the same four decades, cure rates for adult cancer have barely shifted. That is despite President Nixon's 1970 declaration that he was directing America to declare war on the disease.*

The effort that has been put into working out how best to treat childhood cancers is unmatched. Such cancers are rare, and their treatment gets concentrated in a small number of specialist centres. These are exactly the sort of academic institutions where clinical trials are most often carried out. There have been other advantages,

---

* The germ warfare site at Camp Detrick, which Merck was involved with while developing streptomycin, was converted to attack cancer as a result.

too. Here is a 2003 judgement on the situation by Robert Wittes in an editorial in the *New England Journal of Medicine*:

> Finally, for reasons that are still obscure, many childhood cancers are very responsive to treatment, and cure has long been both a feasible objective for treatment and a powerful motivator of physicians' behavior. As a consequence of this alignment of favorable tumor biology with a culture oriented toward cooperative clinical research, the majority of children with cancer in the United States receive definitive treatment for cancer while enrolled in clinical trials. The benefits have been monumental; the curability of most cancer in childhood stands as one of the great success stories of modern medicine.

The editorial points out that adult cancers are common by comparison. Treatments for them are less successful, so doctors have not got into a virtuous circle of being so encouraged by the innovations of the year before that they plunge into fresh ones. As a result of all of this, the vast majority of adult cancer patients are *not* treated within clinical trials. Although their numbers provide plentiful opportunities for research, there has never been the same degree of interest. Robert Wittes, writing the *New England Journal* editorial, was clearly as angry about this failure for adults as he was delighted with the success for children:

> Of the many things that physicians do, participating in cooperative clinical trials is among the strangest. Relatively undervalued in the typical academic promotion-and-tenure process, often inadequately reimbursed by government funding agencies, faced with informed-consent regulations that vastly exceed in degree of disclosure what is required for routine care, and confronting progressively greater degrees of regulation

with each passing year, the clinical trialist may be forgiven for occasionally wondering whether society really wants this kind of work to go forward.

Leaving aside his complaints about the difficulties of performing clinical trials, what about their ethics? Are children within trials, who get allocated to the older treatments, sacrificing their lives for the benefits of medical progress? Have the wonderful advances in treatment for childhood cancer been bought at the expense of children who entered the trials and did not get the latest therapies?

New treatments do not get tried on children (or adults) without a great deal of testing beforehand. Trial treatments are ones that researchers think *should* work. The theory supporting them is excellent. If they are drugs, then in laboratory studies, in test tubes and on cell cultures, they will have shown benefit. They will have been tried on animals, to test both their safety and their effectiveness. An initial small trial will have been done on humans, to check the drug's immediate impact and toxicity. If the results are acceptable a second trial – phase II – will be carried out, to see if the safety and effectiveness from animal studies appear to carry through into human children. Only if the drug still looks good at this stage will a phase III trial be carried out. This is usually a full-blown, randomised, controlled, double-blinded effort to find out exactly what the drug's effects in people are. After all the testing that goes on before it starts, it is almost impossible to believe that those allocated to the latest treatment will not be better off than those who volunteer to enter the trial but get used as controls. Why then should any sick child submit to being part of a such a trial, and risk being used as a control?

The common perception of the situation was summed up by Henry Waxman, an American member of Congress talking to CNN in 1995. 'I think that both with regard to AIDS and cancer and any other life-threatening disease,' he said, 'we ought to make available to people as quickly as possible drugs and other therapies that may extend their lives and not wait until we know with certainty that something is going to be effective.'

Congressman Waxman's comment expresses the age-old urge to *do something* in the face of illness. It is backed up by a belief in the effectiveness of modern medicine, and a confidence that doctors are now able to come up with powerful new therapies. People in the past may not have known what worked without performing proper tests, but these days our understanding of science is so much more advanced. Maybe today these painstaking tests are not needed so much, and the Congressman was right that withholding new treatments while they undergo rigorous examination is cruel. Some people, after all, will die before the trials are finished.

In response to these concerns, a group of researchers led by Ambuj Kumar took a thorough look at the history of new childhood cancer treatments, publishing their results in December 2005. They collated a group of 126 different trials performed between 1955 and 1997. Every new treatment they looked at was approved only after strict review procedures. None was the result of individual enthusiasms; they came from the thoughtful opinions of large groups of scientists and doctors. All of the treatments were being tested in high-quality, phase III, randomised, controlled trials.

What the researchers were worried about was whether modern doctors were so good at predicting improved treatments that the kids who got them were likely to be better off. They did not imagine that all the new treatments would turn out to work – there are always some surprises – their concern was that more than half of them might work. If they did, the ethical grounds for doing randomised trials were shaky. If more than half of the new therapies worked, then individual children would always be better off refusing to enter a trial and insisting on whatever the doctors thought was probably going to be best.

Altogether the trials included almost 37,000 children. Some of the new treatments turned out to be breakthroughs. Others, of course, were disappointments, being no better than what came before them. There were even some that, despite all the promising signs that they were going to be helpful, actually caused harm. On average, taking all the trials and all the children, new treatments turned out to be as likely to harm as to help, as likely to be worse as better in comparison to what came before.

That is, with the most advanced molecular underpinnings, the best laboratory scientists, with superb and highly motivated doctors and researchers, extensive trials in cancer models, then in animals, then on a small scale in actual children – with all of this, the greatest cancer experts in the world were unable to predict what worked and what did not without actually doing a trial.

What got the authors of this research most excited was not the fact that this meant that asking children to enter trials posed no ethical problems. What they found inspirational was the way in which childhood cancer researchers had turned their uncertainties into therapeutic victories. 'The success has not come from a series of continuous, steady improvements, as selective reporting of treatment accomplishments may lead us to believe. On the contrary, our data show that outcomes of new treatments are as likely to be inferior as they are to be superior to standard treatments.' The 'successful evolution of treatment resulted from empirical testing by investigators who acknowledged their uncertainty and chose to randomise between treatments, the relative effect of which they could not predict'. When some of the same authors repeated the exercise with a different medical speciality, radiation therapy, collecting together fifty-seven trials on almost 13,000 people, done between 1968 and 2002, the results were the same. Innovative treatments were just as likely to be worse than what came before as they were to be better.

Congressman Waxman was wrong. The more serious the disease, the *more* important it becomes to actually test out what works, to 'wait until we know with certainty that something is going to be effective', as the Congressman said researchers had no need to. Other studies of doctors' ability to predict the outcomes of trials, in surgery and adult cancer and in anaesthetics, have all shown similar results.

The researchers who surveyed the trials were confident about the implications of their work. As Ambuj Kumar and his colleagues wrote:

> Our findings should underpin the continuing need to resolve uncertainty through the randomised comparison of new and standard treatments. Over the past few decades the use of this principle of randomising when uncertain has served children with cancer well . . . The scientific community and the public should be made more aware of how this mechanism underlies advances in clinical medicine.

AIDS activists in America were successful in pushing for 'compassionate modifications' to the trial process. As a result the American trials in the early 1990s for zidovudine – AZT, the first effective anti-AIDS drug – were altered. The drug interferes with an enzyme called reverse transcriptase, used by retroviruses like HIV to insert their genetic material into that of their hosts. At the time it was unclear if AZT helped people who were infected with HIV but were otherwise healthy, people whose immune systems had not yet been destroyed by the virus and did not yet have AIDS. Rather than taking a 'hard' end point – death, or progression to full-blown AIDS – the modified trials took a short cut. They looked at levels of CD4 cells, the essential component of the immune system that HIV gradually attacks. The intention was to get an answer as quickly as possible, so that as few as possible died while waiting for it. Over a short period, AZT increased the numbers of these CD4 cells. That was enough; Americans, influenced by the organised campaigns of AIDS activists, were convinced. The drug was widely adopted for all HIV patients.

A large European trial was continued all the same. This one did look at hard end points, those of death or progression to AIDS. American activists attacked the trial as unethical. Their own demonstration of AZT's effect on CD4 counts, they argued, established that everyone with HIV should be on the drug regardless of how far their disease had progressed. These were sincere, intelligent and educated people making an argument that it was emotionally very difficult to refute. They were arguing that AZT was life-saving and that those unwilling to see where the evidence pointed were killing HIV sufferers by withholding the drug. This was in the days before there was any other drug besides AZT to slow HIV's progression.

In Britain, Ireland and France, the trial of early AZT carried on despite objections. Enough people felt that there was often a difference between where evidence points and what it eventually shows; a difference between soft outcomes that give some sign of what a disease is doing, and the hard outcomes that show it for certain.

The European trial was published in 1994. It showed that AZT, a drug with significant side effects and to which HIV could rapidly develop resistance, did nothing to increase the survival of HIV-positive patients in the early stage of the disease, or to slow their progression to AIDS. The American optimism was the result of an earnest desire that a drug should help, not a thorough examination of whether it actually did. It turned out to be wrong.

The push from AIDS activists to shortcut lengthy trials continued. Another drug, dideoxyinosine, was released under what was called a 'parallel track'. As well as being used for a clinical trial, in comparison with the existing AZT, it was also released to those outside the trial who wanted to take it. The effects were predictable. Many people were happy to take the drug without definite proof that it worked, judging that it was more likely to do them good than harm. And there were so few left who were willing to be uncertain, that the trial almost collapsed for lack of participants. 'The current turn of events reminds us', wrote a medical commentator at the time, 'that we cannot obtain highly reliable evidence about a new treatment without the full co-operation of relatively large numbers of suffering human beings.' AIDS patients found it difficult to co-operate. Their prejudice that new drugs were likely to work was too strong.

The scepticism that many doctors have so slowly and painfully acquired is not something widely shared outside the profession. Yet the idea that even the most reasonable-sounding theories should be subjected to tests probably has more potential to make the world a better place than all the drugs that doctors possess. Economics, politics, social care and education are full of policies that are based on beliefs held as a matter of principle rather than because they are supported by objective tests. Humility, even more than pills, is the healthiest thing that doctors have to offer.

24   Revolutionary Confidence

Sometimes, when two strong and opinionated men do battle, it is best to be standing well clear. At a distance of a little over two centuries, we are well placed to relish the explosive collision of William Cobbett and Benjamin Rush.

Rush came into the world at Christmas 1745, a little way outside of Philadelphia. Brought up by an evangelistic and hard-working mother, he went into medicine at the age of fifteen. Having already graduated from the College of New Jersey (now Princeton), he studied with leading Philadelphia doctors. The College of Philadelphia, founded in 1749 by Benjamin Franklin, was the first medical school on American shores, but even in the eyes of the most partisan patriots it was not the pinnacle of medical science. Rush studied there and then moved on. For two years from 1766, he was at Edinburgh, the leading medical school in the English-speaking world. He completed his studies with stints in Paris and London before returning to Philadelphia, where he was promptly appointed professor.

Within five years of returning to America Rush was well established, as a politician as well as a doctor. An early abolitionist, he campaigned against slavery in person and print. Thomas Paine's successful 1776 pamphlet *Common Sense*, which did so much to promote the American Revolution, was encouraged, edited and named by Rush. The same year, aged thirty, Rush was elected to the

Second Congressional Congress, signed the Declaration of Independence (chiefly written by his friend Thomas Jefferson), and married the sixteen-year-old daughter of another signatory.

During the subsequent war, Rush showed his willingness to risk his life and lose his friends over issues of conscience. Attached to the Continental army, he provided medical support at many of the major battles. It was at Trenton that 'for the first time war appeared to me in its awful plenitude of horrors'. Thereafter he was at Princeton (where he found friends dying on both sides of the conflict), Brandywine and Germantown. He was with the army during its winter rest in Valley Forge. When Rush wrote to Washington, complaining of the manner in which John Shippen – Rush's old teacher from Philadelphia, now surgeon-general – was organising the army's medical services, Shippen was sacked and court-martialled. Soon afterwards Rush wrote to Patrick Henry, governor of Virginia, suggesting that Washington too was incompetent and ought to be removed from his command. This time Rush came off worst. He left the army and returned home. His next war began in 1793, when yellow fever invaded Philadelphia.

William Cobbett was there at the same time, having arrived by a very different route. 'I do not remember the time when I did not earn my living,' he wrote. 'My first occupation was driving the birds from the turnip-seeds, and the rooks from the peas.' At the time he was barely big enough to make it over a country stile. Later, in 1774 at the ripe age of eleven, Cobbett decided that he wished to work at the Royal Botanical Gardens at Kew, on the edge of London. His decision to go to Kew was impulsive. The eleven-year-old Cobbett set off from his father's farm in Farnham, Surrey, and walked the thirty-five miles to Kew Gardens near Richmond. His unexpected profits from the adventure came when he rashly spent his pennies, not on food, but on a book. 'The title was so odd that my curiosity was excited. I had the threepence, but then I could have no supper.'

Cobbett chose the book and went hungry. It was *A Tale of a Tub*, Jonathan Swift's satire on religion, medicine, politics, and oppression. That first reading of it became, according to Cobbett's later accounts of himself, 'what I have always considered a birth of intellect'. When a later impulse took him into the army nine years later, he used his free time to pursue his love of reading. Posted to Canada, he became a self-educated and forcibly angry sergeant major, provoked by the corruption and injustice around him. After collecting evidence of embezzlement, Cobbett discovered that the officers he was trying to bring to justice were manoeuvring to destroy the evidence and have him framed for treason. He fled to Paris in March 1792, taking his new wife with him. For six months there he was happy, but the Revolutionary bloodshed and the prospect of a war with Britain caused him to flee once again. This time he chose America.

He ended up in Philadelphia. In 1793 it was the nation's capital. Including the suburbs that surrounded it, it was also the largest city, thronged with 40 or even 50,000 souls. Medical opinions were easily gained and, if you wanted someone who held a degree in the subject, you had eighty fully qualified physicians to choose from.

Benjamin Rush, one of them, was the first to suggest that 1793 was seeing a yellow fever epidemic. A feverish illness, characterised by fatal bleeding in many of those affected, it is now known to be a virus spread by certain mosquitoes. From July 1793 it was striking people down on Philadelphia's squalid waterfront. They tended to be the poorest and the most destitute. Their deaths attracted little attention. In August, Rush began seeing cases amongst his own patients. They prompted him to ask his colleagues about their own recent experiences. On hearing that yellow fever was becoming widespread, Rush began pointing out that things were likely to get worse. His views were unpopular. Rush 'was immediately ridiculed and attacked from all sides as an alarmist'. That was despite the fact the city had been struck many times before, from 1699 through to 1762. Fortunately, unpopularity did not scare Dr Rush; he was accustomed to it. He gathered infamy as well as admiration in the course of his many missions, as eager to change people and as willing to fight them as Cobbett. Prison reform, free schooling for the poor, women's rights and kind treatment for the mentally sick – many of Rush's causes were noble. Their desirability, not their practicality, was what appealed to him. If something was right, it was worth pushing for, even if there was no real prospect of success. You never knew until you tried. 'As the War Office of the United States was established in the time of peace,' Rush declared during one of his campaigns, 'it is equally reasonable that a Peace Office should be established in the time of war.' It never has been.

Despite Rush's training at Edinburgh, London and Paris, he felt European doctrines were not suited to America. Old theories seemed to lack power in the New World. Medicine seemed not as effective, and medical beliefs not so accurate, as he had been taught to believe. Like many before him, Rush leapt from this potentially promising realisation into disaster. Rather than questioning the values of theories, and exploring better ways to test them, he came up with his own.

His favourite concerned fever. Rather than representing different diseases, as he had been taught, Rush felt that fever *was* disease. Clearly, he decided, it was something to do with the blood, which was hot. 'I have formerly said there is but one fever in the world. Be not startled, gentlemen, follow me and I will say there is but one disease in the world.' In itself, Rush's theory was neither more effective nor more useless than those of the Scots, English and French who had trained him. In some ways it was not that different either. What mattered was the way he put it into practice.

When yellow fever had last gripped Philadelphia, in 1762, Rush was in his first year at medical school, too inexperienced to form much of an impression. Things were different now. Of the first five patients that Rush saw with yellow fever, four died. Their treatment had been, by contemporary standards, fairly benign. They were given a little mercury to encourage urination and diarrhoea (both of which made them less likely to survive). Then another laxative, to encourage a bit more diarrhoea (worsening their dehydration). Finally, as though to compensate for their medical treatment a little, they were given some food and drink.

Four of the five dying struck Rush as unconscionable. God, he felt, was always willing to provide a cure if only there was someone pious and energetic enough to seek it out. Aflame to do so, Rush read everything he could on yellow fever. He found an account from a doctor working in Virginia, fifty years before. Cutting open his patients after they died, their physician reported that their guts had been full of blood.

Rush had an epiphany. A fever was caused by blood, too much of it. Yellow fever was characterised by people's blood spilling out of them – from their noses and gums, from small wounds and internally into bruises and into their guts. They were obviously dying from an excess of blood! The way forward was clear and he had the pioneering spirit to blaze it.

> I preferred frequent and small, to large bleedings in the beginnings of September, but toward the height and close of the epidemic, I saw no inconvenience from the loss of a pint and even 20 ounces of blood at a time. I drew from many persons 70 and 80 ounces in five days, and from a few a much larger quantity.

Eighty ounces works out at about 2.5 litres, roughly half of the amount of blood within a man's body, and more of a woman's. Rush said that he never once lost a patient that he was able to bleed on seven different occasions. A commentator has pointed out that this was not surprising, given that blood was generally taken on a daily basis and yellow fever worked itself out within seven to ten days. One might also have reasonably observed that anyone able to survive seven encounters with Dr Rush was not going to be snuffed out by anything so mild as a major infective illness.

People fled Philadelphia. Up to half of them left the city while the epidemic was under way. One was Thomas Jefferson, who reckoned that a third of those who picked up the infection quickly died of it. A painstaking modern attempt to find out what happened to Rush's patients suggested that their chances were significantly worse. Only around half survived.

Never anything other than courageous, and committed to trying to make the world a better place in the ways he saw open to him, Rush refused to quit his post. That put him in a minority, and a dangerous one. Of the doctors who stayed, ten died. At one point there were only two others, besides Rush, left living in the city. The worse the disease got, the more Rush's conviction grew that he held in his hands the power to save people. 'Americans are tougher than Europeans,' taught Rush. 'American diseases are, correspondingly, tougher than mild European diseases; to cure Americans will require uniquely powerful doses administered by heroic American physicians.' He increased tenfold the doses of mercury and of laxatives that he gave to his patients. He recommended that the majority of their blood be removed, up to 80 per cent of what they contained. When he felt ill himself, one day in September, he swallowed some laxatives and had a colleague remove over a pint of blood. The next day he felt better and returned to tending the sick. Their blood covered the front yard of Rush's house, and the flies swarmed to it. 'Never before', said Rush, 'did I experience such a sublime joy as I now felt in contemplating the success of my remedies.' In the hundred days that yellow fever besieged the depopulated city, over 4,000 of those who remained died.

When the epidemic finished, Rush's joy continued. His theories were proven and his powers demonstrated. 'Depletion therapy', as it was called, became something that Rush evangelised. It worked for pretty much everything, he explained, but it was especially good for yellow fever. Since Philadelphia went on to have annual epidemics over the next few years, he had reason to do everything he could to persuade people of the value of his discovery.

Rush burnt with a sense of mission. Part of it came from his sense of religious duty, the rest from his conviction that the New World offered an opportunity – practically required a duty – for forward-thinking men to conquer the limitations of the natural world. Other doctors placed 'undue reliance upon the powers of nature in curing disease'. Action, felt Rush, was what was needed, a willingness to practise in medicine what the new Americans were doing in politics, a willingness to be 'heroic, bold, courageous, manly, and patriotic'.

Oliver Wendell Holmes later described Rush's position with damning sympathy:

His mind was in a perpetual state of exaltation produced by the stirring scenes in which he had taken part . . . But he could not help feeling that Nature had been a good deal shaken by the Declaration of Independence, and that American [medical] art was getting to be rather too much for her – especially as illustrated in his own practice.

William Cobbett, writing about the yellow fever epidemics from 1793 onwards, was not so charitable. 'Bleeding a man to death, no matter what the disease,' he suggested, 'could not be the proper method of saving his life.' The actions of Rush appalled him, and wielding his satirical newspaper, the *Porcupine's Gazette*, he rode into battle. There is no doubt that part of Cobbett's anger was due to Rush's political beliefs, and the doctor's tendency, like Jefferson, to overlook the worst parts of the French Revolution in order to praise its ideals. Having watched the slaughter in Paris at first hand, Cobbett was in no mood to keep quiet while another needless massacre took place. And if Rush was skilled at drawing blood with a lancet, so was Cobbett with his pen.

In this case the truth, as well as the louder voice, belonged to Cobbett. The *Porcupine's Gazette* 'was the most widely read newspaper in the United States'. That was quite an achievement for a publication whose editor was patriotically English, and whose stingingly satiric views were English to match. Even George Washington read it, and sent copies to friends. 'Making allowances for the asperity of an Englishman,' he said to one, 'for some of his strong and coarse expressions; and a want of official information of many facts; it is not a bad thing.'

Cobbett mocked Rush's use of mercury and accused him of ensuring that tens of thousands of American lives were lost through poisoning and blood loss. 'The mode of treatment advised by Doctor Rush cannot, in the yellow fever, fail of being certain death,' he wrote. A libel suit followed. It was brought by Rush in the autumn of 1797. The court hearing, however, was extensively delayed – possibly due to other enemies of Rush, keen to prolong and publicise his ordeal.

Cobbett's attacks successfully destroyed Rush as a doctor; they failed to accomplish the better alternative of improving him. Jefferson had written to Rush on the importance of tolerance between those who disagreed. 'With a man possessing so many other estimable qualities, why should we be dissocialized by mere difference of opinion in politics, in religion, in philosophy, or anything else?' Despite their mutual zeal for reforming others, this was not a view that appealed much to Cobbett or Rush.

Thursday 12 December was a cold day in Virginia. Washington rode around his farm in rain, hail and snow, then had his evening meal without changing his wet clothes. The next day he felt unwell and spent it quietly, staying mostly indoors. In the evening he read aloud to his wife before going to bed. Between two and three in the morning, Washington woke her to tell her that he felt worse. In the morning, the Saturday, Washington asked his plantation supervisor to bleed him. The man took away around a third of a litre of Washington's blood. Before lunchtime the first doctor arrived. He bled Washington twice more, removing another litre and a quarter litres (over two pints) of blood. When the next doctor arrived in the middle of the afternoon, Washington was bled another full litre. Mercury was given in order to induce diarrhoea. Repeated doses of drugs were used to make Washington vomit. Hot cups were applied to his flesh to raise up large blood-filled blisters.

Washington probably contained about five litres of blood, of which over half was directly removed by bleeding. The vomiting, diarrhoea and blistering helped dehydrate him further, as did the fever and inflammation that came from being unwell in the first place. Towards the end of the Saturday, the physicians now crowding around Washington's bed noticed that his blood seemed different. Rather than flowing with brisk freedom when a vein or an artery was opened, it was thick and sticky and only oozed away slowly.

'Pray take no more trouble about me,' Washington told his doctors. 'Let me go quietly.' He died a little after ten o'clock on the Saturday evening.

Writing the following February, William Cobbett reckoned the total amount of blood removed came to '108 ounces, which is nine pounds, and which makes in measure, nine pints, or one gallon and a pint!!!' He thought it deserved a few exclamation marks. There is every reason to distrust his higher total, but to respect the feelings that led him to inflate it. Washington had successfully brought America into peaceful relations with Britain, fighting off the efforts of the more pro-French republicans like Jefferson. To Cobbett he was something of a hero. And Washington's death was hastened, if not entirely caused, by the attentions of his doctors.

Exacerbating Cobbett's feeling of outrage was the fact that on the same day that Washington died, Rush's libel suit against him was concluded. 'The times are ominous indeed,' Cobbett's lawyer said in court, 'when quack to quack cries purge and bleed.' The judge, a man whom Cobbett had attacked in print years previously, found against him. Rush was awarded damages of $5,000. Cobbett pointed out that this exceeded the combined sum awarded in every similar court case since the United States had been founded. It was enough to make him flee back to Britain to escape.

He lingered long enough before returning, however, to attack the medical care that Washington had received, and to bring evidence as well as opinion to bear on his criticism of Rush. Having abandoned the *Porcupine's Gazette*, his new publication – pointedly called *The Rush-Light* – looked at the official registry of deaths in Philadelphia. After Rush began advertising his belief in heroic levels of bleeding, Cobbett noted, the mortality rate demonstrably rose.

The existence of other people holding different views from ourselves is a problem for all of us. Cobbett and Rush could have come together, recognised that one of them had to be wrong about the effects of bleeding and devised an experiment to settle their differences. Both were idealists, vigorous in their pursuit of many goals they held dear. Neither man doubted his ability to reason out truth without recourse to a test. It happens that Cobbett was right and Rush wrong but their unwillingness to put their beliefs to a trial matters more. 'Ignorance is preferable to error,' wrote Jefferson in his 1782 *Notes on Virginia*, 'and he is less remote from the truth who believes nothing than he who believes what is wrong.' It was a lesson that was not to the tastes of those who felt strong opinions were more manly than uncertainties and doubts.

A few years later, in 1803, Meriwether Lewis came to Rush in order to learn some medicine. He was sent by Jefferson, who wanted to prepare Lewis for his historic journey with William Clark across America to the Pacific North-west. Rush equipped Lewis with a half a pound of opium, drugs to induce vomiting, fifty dozen mercury-based laxative pills, a pound of mercury (to be taken orally or injected directly into the penis in the event of picking up a sexually transmitted disease), fifteen pounds of Peruvian bark and two pounds of an ointment made up of animal fat, beeswax and pine resin. The expedition used so much of Rush's mercury that now, more than two centuries later, their rest stops are identifiable as the earth around the places they used as toilets is still so contaminated.

The moral is not that doctors once did foolish things. The moral is that even the best of people let themselves down when they rely on untested theories, and that these failures kill people and stain history. Bleeding and mercury have gone out of fashion, untested certainties and over-confidence have not.

25   The Beauty of Doubts

To what extent are the things that doctors do today proven to be useful?

When Archie Cochrane interrupted a talk in New Zealand in 1976, to call his friend Kerr White 'a damned liar' for suggesting that any more than 10 per cent of medical interventions were based on good evidence, he was not pulling his statistics out of the Wellington air. The figure came from a 1963 paper in *Medical Care* reporting the results of a fortnight's survey of nineteen family doctors in the north of England. They were asked to keep records of every prescription written over that period, and at the end of the time the drugs they prescribed were compared with the conditions they were trying to treat, and an attempt was made to determine how many were supported by reliable evidence. The figure came out as 9.3 per cent – inflated by Cochrane to a round 10.

Efforts to extend the degree to which medical practice is based on sound evidence have been going on – with stuttering success – throughout human history. The power of randomised controlled trials, and the extent to which most of what doctors did was not backed up by them, became increasingly apparent over the course of the twentieth century. Statistical work establishing the effectiveness of medical interventions was called 'clinical epidemiology' for most of that period. The name came to seem too obscure and off-putting for what was felt to be universally important and relevant. As a result, a different term appeared during the 1980s, emerging from medical teaching sessions at McMaster University in Canada. 'Evidence-based medicine' (EBM) first appears in the literature in a 1991 article in the *Journal of the American Medical Association*. These days the term is widely used. In its mocking tautology, 'evidence-based medicine' is clearly a propaganda term. It is a euphemism for a school of thinking that holds that certain types of evidence are generally more robust and valuable than others – experiments more than guesses, trials more than anecdotes, interventions more than observations.

Many doctors loathe the term 'evidence-based medicine', their hackles raised by its campaigning tone and its implication that they are doing something different. Arguments are frequently made that it is a movement that seeks experimental proof for the most ludicrous of things and in the most thoughtless of ways. A good example is the 2003 *British Medical Journal* paper by Gordon Smith and Jill Pell, entitled 'Parachute Use to Prevent Death and Major Trauma Related to Gravitational Challenge':

> As with many interventions intended to prevent ill health, the effectiveness of parachutes has not been subjected to rigorous evaluation by using randomised controlled trials. Advocates of evidence based medicine have criticised the adoption of interventions evaluated by using only observational data. We think that everyone might benefit if the most radical protagonists of evidence based medicine organised and participated in a double blind, randomised, placebo controlled, crossover trial of the parachute.

In contrast, advocates of EBM seem happy to accept that interventions like parachutes are clearly helpful. A 1995 *Lancet* paper, 'Inpatient general medicine is evidence based', gives a good guide to the standards of evidence that are actually required by 'the most radical protagonists of evidence based medicine', as well as suggesting that medicine has improved since 1963. One of the paper's authors was the Canadian doctor David Sackett, who has been amongst the foremost evangelists for the EBM movement. The paper looked at all the treatments given to patients coming under the care of Sackett's team of physicians in a single month at the John Radcliffe Hospital in Oxford. Sackett commented:*

We found that a service that ran like ours and worked hard to find the best evidence to guide its interventions could treat 53% of its patients on the basis of SRs [systematic reviews bringing together combinations of high-quality trials] and RCTs [Randomised Controlled Trials], another 29% on the basis of convincing non-experimental evidence, and just 19% on the basis of guessing and hope.

Over 80 per cent of decisions being based on good verification is a stunning improvement, even in a medical team led by a physician with an avowed devotion to following evidence. Sackett gave an example of the sort of treatment that he felt did not require randomised controlled evidence before being accepted as true: giving an electric shock to someone's heart when it has stopped beating. In medical terms, such a shock is analogous with using a parachute. There are rare cases of people surviving without either – falling 10,000 feet into trees and snow, or spontaneously having their heart recover a normal rhythm – but in general the intervention, be it a parachute or an electric shock, is required for survival.

The study sparked off a series of similar surveys in different medical settings and specialities. Two looked at the evidence base within the world of family doctors. The first, a study from Leeds

---

* See www.shef.ac.uk/Scharr/in/percent.html

(Gill *et al.*) was published in the *British Medical Journal* in 1996. Two days' worth of consultations within a single family practice came up with similar figures to the *Lancet* paper, with 31 per cent of treatments being based on RCT evidence and 51 per cent on 'convincing non-experimental evidence'. The same year, and also in the *British Medical Journal*, a group of Japanese family doctors led by Koki Tsuruoka reported the results of reviewing forty-nine of their own consultations (around half the number of both the Oxford and the Leeds study). Using the same criteria for deciding on what was convincing proof as the other two studies, they found that 81 per cent of their treatments were based on good evidence.

Repeating the 1995 *Lancet* study in Kyoto University Hospital, Hiroshi Koyama and colleagues looked at how many of their treatment decisions were based on RCT evidence. Writing in the *International Journal for Quality in Health Care* in 2002, they looked at 211 different therapeutic interventions, finding 49 per cent of them to be supported specifically by RCTs, roughly the same as for Sackett's hospital team in Oxford.

Other specialities have repeated these efforts to assess the extent to which their practices are based on evidence. In 2006, in a paper in the online journal *BMC Women's Health*, which looked at obstetrics and gynaecology, Aamir Khan and others from Birmingham, England, reviewed 325 consecutive inpatients from 1998 and 1999, finding 42 per cent of the interventions the patients received to be based on RCTs.

A 1998 paper from Great Ormond Street Children's Hospital suggested that contemporary paediatric surgery was less well founded on relevant research. Investigating a month of operations at this leading hospital, Baraldini and other surgeons concluded 26 per cent of seventy operations were founded on RCTs while 3 per cent fell into the category of being self-evidently helpful. That left another 3 per cent whose operations, in retrospect, appeared to go against all available evidence and 68 per cent without any adequate evidence base either way. An audit by ophthalmic surgeons in Hong Kong (Lai *et al.*), published in 2003 in the *British Journal of Ophthalmology*, found that 43 per cent of their 274 consecutive interventions in July 2002 were supported by RCTs, 34 per cent had the backing of poorer-quality observational evidence, and the remaining 23 per cent were either unsupported by any evidence whatsoever, or contradicted by it.

Other measurements of the extent to which medicine is now evidence-based have been similar to those given in the papers above. It is clear that we can be more confident in medical therapeutics today than we were in 1963; it is not only that our treatments have improved, it is also that we now have a much more certain knowledge of what their real effects are.

What about the estimates that some of these trials made of treatments that were 'obviously' true? What did they decide was so self-evident that it required no RCT evidence? The Kyoto team of Hiroshi Koyama declared forty-seven treatments to fit in this category, including (as at Oxford) the example of delivering an electric shock to someone after their heart has stopped. They also listed removing an appendix in a patient with appendicitis, giving oxygen to people in respiratory difficulty, watchful inactivity for those with glandular fever, blood-thinning with warfarin for people with deep-vein thromboses and the administration of insulin or thyroid hormones to those whose bodies have stopped producing them.

The 1996 family doctor study from Leeds (Gill *et al.*) also included giving thyroid hormones in their list of forty-three 'interventions substantiated by convincing non-experimental evidence'. Other remedies seem similarly clear, like fluids for those who are dehydrated. But their list also included therapies that appear more immediately questionable, such as a range of specific antibiotics for particular infections. Some of these, like tonsillitis and chest infections, are likely to be viral rather than bacterial in origin – and although the antibiotics they mentioned were ones that are very safe, they, like all drugs, still sometimes have harms. (It is a reliable generalisation that the only drug with no side effects is one that does nothing at all.) Strong painkillers for back pain were also listed as unarguably good. This is likely to be true but, given that gentler analgesics might provide useful benefits with lower risks of serious harms (such as gastro-intestinal bleeding), it is questionable.

Contemporary mistakes about medical knowledge seem to come from two main directions. The first is the failure to properly test a hypothesis because it seems so obviously true. An excellent recent example is that of hormone replacement therapy (HRT). For decades post-menopausal women took hormones to replace those that their own bodies had stopped producing. The idea that this was good was based on theories of human physiology; it was reasonable to suspect that replacing in old age a set of hormones that were present in youth was helpful. Later, observations showed that women who took replacement hormones after their menopause actually did live longer and enjoy better health than women who did not.

The trouble was that these observations were taken as constituting an experiment. They did not. Women were not being randomly allocated to either taking the hormones or not taking them – they were choosing. That meant it was entirely possible that the sort of women who made one choice were different from those who made another. Nevertheless it took until 1993 for a relevant trial to be set up. The Women's Health Initiative was an American study that enrolled over 160,000 post-menopausal women and allocated them to either HRT or placebo. In 2002 the trial was stopped early after the number of deaths from breast cancer was found to be higher than expected in the group taking HRT. British estimates suggest that HRT use in the UK alone was causing 2,000 extra cases of breast cancer a year. Despite this, the Women's Health Initiative study had not actually been set up to test whether HRT was safe. It was established because doctors believed it would prove that HRT was saving lives.

The second mistake commonly still made is accepting trial evidence of the right kind, but which has not actually been carried out well enough to be reliable. Antidepressants are a good example. There have been hosts of studies, many of them randomised, double-blinded and controlled. But the studies have been undercut by being too small, too short, too badly designed and too vulnerable to being misrepresented by those with vested interests. That such trials continue to be accepted, both by governments and doctors, comes from the failure of both to understand the nature and importance of a good evidence base.

A bad study is clearly untrustworthy, such as those carried out in the early days of thalidomide, which made no serious attempts to objectively assess the drug. When it comes to depression, there are a host of drugs available, many only very slightly different from one another. What we ideally want to know is the precise effect of every one of these drugs compared to every other one, over a long period and in relation to the effects that most matter to people – in this case whether they are helped to be safe, healthy and happy.

Drug companies fund trials only as much as they need in order to persuade doctors to prescribe a treatment and governments to allow it. That leads to problems. A survey of the evidence behind twelve different antidepressants appeared in the *New England Journal of Medicine* in 2008 (Turner *et al.*). It looked at the trial data that drug companies submitted to the FDA when applying for regulatory approval, and compared that to the data that were eventually pub-lished and available for public view. Drug companies are obliged to register clinical studies with the FDA, and to submit results regardless of what they show. They are not obliged to publish them.

The paper found seventy-four relevant studies covering over 12,000 patients. 'Studies viewed by the FDA as having negative or questionable results', said the paper, 'were, with 3 exceptions, either not published (22 studies) or published in a way that, in our opinion, conveyed a positive outcome (11 studies). According to the published literature, it appeared that 94% of the trials conducted were positive. By contrast, the FDA analysis showed that 51% were positive.' The authors felt unable to conclude whether this difference in what was publicly presented – an effect called 'publication bias' – was because drug companies put forward only their most favourable results, or because medical journals were uninterested in printing studies showing treatments had no compelling effects. The drugs approved by the FDA all showed benefit when all relevant results were brought together, but the paper found that these benefits were not accurately presented to the medical profession – 'selective pub- lication', they concluded, 'can lead doctors to make inappropriate prescribing decisions that may not be in the best interest of their patients'. An earlier 2004 paper (by Whittington *et al.*) in the *Lancet* found the same when looking at selective serotonin reuptake inhibitors (SSRIs), a class of antidepressant drug, when used for depression in children. The effectiveness of the drugs appeared quite different when unpublished drug company trials were combined with those that had been published – benefits had appeared to outweigh harms, but adding in the extra data suggested the opposite.

Are these effects important? A 2004 study (by An-Wen Chan and others) in the *Journal of the American Medical Association*, said yes. Chan's team looked at clinical trials approved between 1994 and 1995 in Denmark, then followed up the way they had been presented. Between the time that they received ethical approval and the time they published their results, almost two thirds of trials (62 per cent) changed what it was they said they were chiefly measuring – an excellent way of adjusting any trial to make it reach the conclusion

298

you want. (By statistical convention, a finding is regarded as numerically significant if there is less than one in twenty chance of it happening by luck alone. Therefore for every twenty tests you perform, one is likely to appear positive when it represents nothing other than the play of chance. A good study will declare from the beginning the main thing it is aiming to test, and stick to it.) 'The reporting of trial outcomes is not only frequently incomplete,' found Chan's study, 'but also biased and inconsistent with protocols. Published articles, as well as reviews that incorporate them, may therefore be unreliable and overestimate the benefits of an intervention.' They wanted the regulatory rules changed to force researchers to publish their results in a more accurate and comprehensive manner.

The Cochrane Collaboration was formed to pursue Archie Cochrane's goal of making medicine more evidence-based. A non-governmental organisation with the aim of publishing comprehensive analyses of the available data on different treatments, it has undertaken several reviews of antidepressants. One review published in 2004 paid particular attention to the way in which studies of these drugs might be misleading when compared with *inactive* placebo tablets.* Given that antidepressants cause side effects, it is reasonable to think that many people are able to tell whether they have been given a placebo instead – and since the placebo effect rests on believing that you are not actually taking a placebo, this matters. Three Cochrane Collaboration reviewers looked at trials that specifically used an 'active' placebo in order to overcome this, a placebo designed to produce similar side effects to the active drug with none of the main effects. (They were looking at studies of a class

---

* There has been relatively little effort made to compare different antidepressants with each other, an expensive business that drug companies do not voluntarily pursue. That they fail to do suggests that they have little conviction that any one agent is better than another, as well as being a reminder that governments do nothing to demand such studies.

of antidepressants called tricyclics that commonly cause effects like a dry mouth, dry nose and constipation.) The review found nine such studies, containing a total of 751 patients, and showing much smaller than expected differences between the active placebos and the tricyclics. 'This suggests that unblinding effects may inflate the efficacy of antidepressants in trials using inert placebos,' they concluded. The bulk of the good properties that antidepressants were believed to have, in other words, were probably fictional – reflecting only the consequence of carrying out badly designed studies.

Early in 2008, a paper was published that drew widespread attention to the issue of whether antidepressants do far less than most doctors and patients believe (Kirsch *et al.*). Perhaps one of the most curious aspects of the paper, was that much of what it had to say was not new. Irving Kirsch, of the Department of Psychology at the University of Hull, had published a very similar study in 2002 while at the University of Connecticut. Then he had looked at the data submitted to the FDA for approval of the six most popular antidepressants between 1987 and 1999. He found that almost all (80 per cent) of the drugs' beneficial effects came from their power as a placebo. The 20 per cent left over appeared to be definitely there, but not necessarily to matter very much. On the Hamilton Depression Scale, the method commonly accepted for measuring depression, it made a difference of about 2 points. In Britain the National Institute for Clinical Excellence (NICE), a governmental body set up to independently assess the effectiveness and safety of medical interventions, set a cut-off of 3 points as being clinically useful. (An effect can be statistically measurable but too small to be worthwhile to a patient, particularly if it comes at the expense of a known chance of side effects.) Kirsch's 2008 study looked at four of the newer antidepressants, and attempted to see if they were particularly effective or ineffective in relation to the severity of someone's depression. It found the drugs made a similar difference overall, again less than the minimum that NICE believed was genuinely useful. Among the small minority of patients who were most severely depressed, the difference was slightly larger. The fact that their 2008 study drew the bulk of its public attention for findings that were already in their 2002 paper shows another problem: disseminating information can be as difficult as gathering it to begin with.

There are worse things than the widespread use of generally ineffective drugs. Antidepressants are not a scandal like the poisonous elixir of sulphonamide, or thalidomide. But they are a reminder that regulatory frameworks currently fail to make sure that, as doctors or as patients, we have the information we need about the full impacts of many medical interventions.

In the past regulatory reforms have usually followed on from the sort of tragedies that do leave people dead or permanently disabled. Currently we have the opportunity to improve them voluntarily, without waiting for the next medical catastrophe to come to light and force us into action.

The story of our development of testing is a tale of mental advances that have showered riches upon the world, and are hardly known about.

Testing and experiment and trial have always been a part of human life, and their failure to protect us from deluded cures and poisonous remedies tells us something vital. They cannot be relied upon unless they have sufficient method to them, and the quality of that method determines the quality of their results. It is not enough to use words like 'test' and 'experiment' and 'trial' without understanding that they can mean something no better than a guess, or something so organised and reliable as a double-blind, randomised, controlled trial.

Paying attention to the errors that those before us have made, noticed and reported can be profoundly useful. Not only is our understanding of their care and trouble deepened, but our chance of repeating their mistakes is a little reduced. Historians often argue that it is 'sympathetic' to view people the way they viewed themselves, and to look for ways of excusing them for not doing better than they did. That seems to me a condescending approach. Those who thought seriously about how to help their sick fellows were not trying to do 'as well as could be expected'. They did not mean for their theories to be 'perfectly reasonable given the way people understood the world at the time'. They meant to do their patients some good and to uncover the truth, and we take them most seriously when we recognise the ways they often failed.

In his book *Effectiveness & Efficiency*, first published in 1971, Archie Cochrane wrote:

> Two of the most striking changes in word usage in the last twenty years are the upgrading of 'opinion' in comparison with other types of evidence, and the downgrading of the word 'experiment'. The upgrading of 'opinion' has doubtless many causes, but one of the most potent is, I am sure, the television interviewer and producer. They want everything to be brief, dramatic, black and white. Any discussion of evidence is written off as lengthy, dull, and grey. I have seldom heard a television interviewer ask anyone what his evidence was for some particular statement.

Lewis Thomas was born in 1913, four years after Cochrane, and qualified at Harvard Medical School in 1937. Despite sulphonamides, he found contemporary hospitals offered little more to the sick than hotel accommodation. 'Whether you survived or not depended on the natural history of the disease itself,' he wrote. 'Medicine made little or no difference.'

Bad as things were, when he looked back at his father's medical training, he was impressed at how much they had improved. A quarter of a century before him, his father had qualified from Columbia. The cutting-edge training that Thomas's father received contained far more truth about the human body than had ever been known before. By the start of the twentieth century, knowledge of the sciences underpinning medicine was full of sophistication – in pathology, microbiology, physiology, chemistry and even pharmacology. In practice, however, medicine was scarcely different from how it had been for thousands of years. 'Paper after paper', found Thomas when he looked at his father's books, 'recounts the benefits of bleeding, cupping, violent purging, the raising of blisters by vesicant ointments, the immersion of the body in either ice water or intolerably hot water . . . Endless lists of botanical extracts cooked up and mixed together under the influence of nothing more than pure whim.' It is strange what people were, and were not, capable of. At the same time as Galen was recommending ineffective potions and leeches, the Romans were performing architectural and engineering marvels. By the time Thomas's father was being taught largely identical potions and leeches, Einstein had his theory of relativity and aeroplanes were taking to the skies.

What was missing in medicine was experimental method. People could apply it to the hard sciences, but doctors believed in the power of their intuition. They relied on trial and error, and in such an unstructured way that it was of little use. As Lewis Thomas wrote:

> My first hope is for removal of substantial parts of the curriculum in the first two years, making enough room for a few courses in medical ignorance, so that students can start out with a clear view of the things medicine does not know.

There is a bitter joke in modern medicine: the violence with which someone makes an argument is inversely proportional to the amount of evidence they have backing it up. The more people are left without reliable experiments, the more they seem to fall back on strongly held opinions, as though confidence was a starch that could stiffen ideas into facts simply by being applied with enough fervour.

History shows that there is a better way of behaving. What could do us more good than understanding that many of our opinions can be tested, and that those which *can* be tested *should* be tested? The medical mistakes of the past tell us that beliefs based on theories that are untestable, or simply yet to be tested, need to be held humbly. Randomised controlled trials have swept away much suffering and error from hospitals and homes, ushering in comfort and healing instead. Trials can be full of statistics; difficult to understand and laborious to undertake. They have a loveliness to them all the same, and it comes from their power to uncover parts of the reality we live in.

It seems to be our nature to prefer credulity to doubt, confidence to scepticism. We share a tendency to simplify and confuse things, to slip into mental habits that let us down. But by acknowledging this we can be on our guard against it. When it comes to certain questions about the world, questions where the possible answers can be experimentally tested, 'scientific' becomes synonymous with 'rational'. Without demanding evidence, without understanding the qualities that make it reliable, we are vulnerable.

Within the medical profession, many people feel threatened by the rise of clinical trials. They are frightened by the statistics, or by the feeling that others understand such numbers better than they. A clinical trial, these people say, will not replace the rich complexity of an interaction between a patient and a doctor. Yet no one ever suggested it could, or should. Trials tell you certain truths about the world, but not others. They add to your ability to make decisions. They do not wipe out the importance of making them.

The technique of the randomised controlled trial has a splendour to it, as do the parts of human life to which it is wholly inapplicable.

No statistical test or trial design will help tell you if you are in love, or if you are loved in return. That does not mean that trials and statistics are useless, only that they have their place. That place is a fine one. Experiments and numbers reveal truths: they are tools for understanding the world, and for making it better.

Bibliography

Alderson, Philip and Roberts, Ian, 'Corticosteroids in acute traumatic brain injury', *British Medical Journal* 314 1855–1859 (1997)

Altman, Lawrence K., 'The Doctor's World: Little-Known Doctor Who Found New Use for Common Aspirin', *New York Times*, 9 July 1991

American Journal of Public Health, 'Sanocrysin – A Gold Cure for Tuberculosis', (February 1925): 144–5

Aubrey, John, *Brief Lives*, Ann Arbor, 1962

Baraldini, V. *et al.*, 'Evidence-based Operations in Paediatric Surgery', *Paediatric Surgery International* 13, 5–6 (July 1998): 331–5

Bastian, H., *Down and Almost out in Scotland: George Orwell, Tuberculosis and Getting Streptomycin in 1948*, 2004; the James Lind Library: www.jameslindlibrary.org [accessed Thursday 5 October 2007]

Bell, Robert, *Impure Science*, Wiley, 1992

Beral, Valerie, 'Ovarian Cancer and Hormone Replacement Therapy in the Million Women Study', *The Lancet* 369 (2007): 1703–10

Braithwaite, William, *The Retrospect of Medicine*, vol. XLII (July–December), London, Simpkin, 1860

Brownstein, Michael, 'A Brief History of Opiates, Opioid Peptides, and Opioid Receptors', *Proc. Natl. Acad. Sci. USA* 90 (June 1993), 5391–3

Brynner, Rock and Stephens, Trent, *Dark Remedy*, 2001

Burt, C., 'Francis Galton and His Contributions to Psychology', *British Journal of Statistical Psychology* 15 (1962): 1–49

Carnwath, Tom and Smith, Tom, *Heroin Century*, 2002

CAST Investigators, 'Preliminary Report: Effect of Encainide and Flecainide on Mortality', *New England Journal of Medicine* 321, 6 (10 August 1989): 406–12

Chalmers, Iain, 'What is the Prior Probability of a Proposed New Treatment Being Superior to Established Treatments?', *British Medical Journal* (1997): 314 (7073): 74–5

Chalmers, Iain, *MRC Therapeutic Trials Committee's Report on Serum Treatment of Lobar Pneumonia, BMJ 1934*, 2002; the James Lind Library: www.jameslindlibrary.org [accessed Monday 8 October 2007]

Chan, An-Wen *et al.*, 'Empirical Evidence for Selective Reporting of Outcomes in Randomized Trials', *Journal of the American Medical Association* 291, 20 (2004) 2457–65

Cobbett, William, *Rural Rides*, ed. and intro. George Woodcock, 1973

Cochrane, Archibald, *Effectiveness & Efficiency*, 1999

Cochrane, Archibald and Blythe, Max, *One Man's Medicine*, 1989

Colebrook, Leonard, 'The Prevention of Puerperal Sepsis'. *Journal of Obstetrics and Gynaecology of the British Empire* 43 (1936): 691–714

Colebrook, Leonard, 'Prontosil in Streptococcal Infections'. *Lancet* 1 (1936): 1441

Colebrook, Leonard, 'The Story of Puerperal Fever – 1800–1950', *British Medical Journal* 1 (1956): 247–252

CRASH study guidelines: http://www.crash.lshtm.ac.uk/ [accessed 23 March 2008]

Crofton, John, *The MRC Randomised Trial of Streptomycin and Its Legacy: a view from the Clinical Front Line*, 2004; the James Lind Library: www.jameslindlibrary.org [accessed Wednesday 18 October 2007]

Davies, Nicholas, Davies, Garland and Sanders, Elizabeth, 'William Cobbett, Benjamin Rush, and the Death of General Washington', *Journal of the American Medical Association* 249, 7 (18 February 1983) 912–5

Diaz, M. and Neuhauser, D., *Lessons from Using Randomization to Assess Gold Treatment for Tuberculosis*, 2004; the James Lind Library:

www.jameslindlibrary.org [accessed Friday 12 October 2007

Diggins, F. W. E., 'The True History of the Discovery of Penicillin', *British Journal of Biomedical Science* 56, 2 (1999): 83–93

Doll, Richard, 'Controlled Trials: the 1948 Watershed', *British Medical Journal* 317 (1998): 1217–20

Dormandy, Thomas, *The Worst of Evils*, 2006

Donaldson, I. M. L., *Ambroise Paré's account in the Oeuvres of 1575 of new methods of treating gunshot wounds and burns*, 2004; the James Lind Library: www.jameslindlibrary.org [accessed Friday 12 October 2007]

Doyle, D., *Eponymous doctors associated with Edinburgh, part 2*, Journal of the Royal College of Physicians of Edinburgh 2006; 36: 374–81

Ellis, J. *et al.*, 'Inpatient General Medicine is Evidence Based', *Lancet* 346, 8972 (12 August 1995): 407–10

Evelyn, John, *Diary and Correspondence*, ed. William Bray (1882)

Farewell, Vern, Johnson, Tony and Armitage, Peter, '"A Memorandum on the Present Position and Prospects of Medical Statistics and Epidemiology" by Major Greenwood', *Statistics in Medicine* 25 (2006) 2161–2177

Forsyth, G., 'An Enquiry into the Drug Bill', *Med. Care* 1 (1963): 10–16

Galton, Francis, 'Statistical Inquiries into the Efficacy of Prayer', *Fortnightly Review* 12 (1872): 125–35

Galton, Francis, *Memories of My Life*, 1908

Gardner, Walter Myers (ed.), *The British Coal-Tar Industry*, 1915

Garfield, Simon, *Mauve*, 2000

Gill, P. *et al.*, 'Evidence Based General Practice', *British Medical Journal* 312 (1996): 819–21

Gillies, Donald, *Artificial Intelligence and Scientific Method*, 1996

Griffin, John Parry and O'Grady, John (eds), *The Textbook of Pharmaceutical Medicine*, 2006

Guyatt, Gordon, 'Evidence-based Medicine', *ACP Journal Club (Annals of Internal Medicine)* 14, supplement 2 (1991): A-16

Hager, Thomas, *The Demon Under the Microscope*, 2006

Hardern, R. D. *et al.*, 'How Evidence Based are Therapeutic Decisions Taken on a Medical Admissions Unit?', *Emergency Medicine Journal* 20 (2003): 447–8

Harvie, David, *Limeys*, 2002

Hawthorne, Fran, *Inside the FDA*, 2005

Heatley, Norman, *Penicillin and Luck*, 2004

Hill, Austin Bradford, *Principles of Medical Statistics*, 1937

Hill, Austin Bradford, 'The Environment and Disease: Association or Causation?', *Proceedings of the Royal Society of Medicine* 58 (1965): 295–300

Hill, Austin Bradford and Butler, William, 'Obituary: Major Greenwood', *Journal of the Royal Statistical Society* 112, Series A (General) (1949): 487–9

Holland, John, *The History and Description of Fossil Fuel, the Collieries and Coal Trade of Great Britain*, 1841

Holmes, Oliver Wendell, *Medical Essays*, 1842

Honigsbaum, Mark, *The Fever Trail*, 2001

Howes, N. *et al.*, 'Surgical Practice is Evidence Based', *British Journal of Surgery* 84, 9 (1997): 1220–3

IMPACT Research Group, 'International Mexiletine and Placebo Antiarrhythmic Coronary Trial (IMPACT)', *European Heart Journal* 7, 9 (1986): 749–59

Ingrams, Richard, *The Life and Adventures of William Cobbett*, 2006

Jefferson, Tom, *Why the MRC Randomized Trials of Whooping Cough (Pertussis) Vaccines Remain Important 40 Years after They Were Done* 2006; the James Lind Library: www.jameslindlibrary.org [accessed Monday 9 July 2007]

Jeffreys, Diarmuid, *Aspirin: The Story of a Wonder Drug*, 2004

Kaptchuk, T., *Early Use of Blind Assessment in a Homoeopathic Scientific Experiment*, 2004; the James Lind Library: www.jameslindlibrary.org [accessed Wednesday 24 October 2007]

Keeble, Thomas, 'A Cure for the Ague: the Contribution of Robert

Talbor', *Journal of the Royal Society of Medicine* 90 (1997): 285–90

Khan, Aamir *et al.*, 'Is General Inpatient Obstetrics and Gynaecology Evidence-based?', *BMC Women's Health* 6 (2006): http://www.bio medcentral.com/1472-6874/6/5

Khan, M. I. Gabriel, *Encyclopedia of Heart Diseases*, 2005

Kingston, W., 'Streptomycin, Shatz v. Waksman, and the Balance of Credit for Discovery', *Journal of the History of Medicine and Allied Sciences* 60, 2 (April 2005): 218–20

Kirsch, Irving *et al.*, 'The Emperor's New Drugs: An Analysis of Antidepressant Medication Data Submitted to the U.S. Food and Drug Administration', *Prevention & Treatment* 5, 1 (July 2002)

Kirsch, Irving *et al.*, 'Initial Severity and Antidepressant Benefits: A Meta-Analysis of Data Submitted to the Food and Drug Administration', *PLoS Medicine* 5, 2 (2008): e45 doi:10.1371/journal.pmed.0050045

Koyama, Hiroshi *et al.*, 'In-patient Interventions Supported by Results of Randomized Controlled Trials in Japan', *International Journal for Quality in Health Care* 14, 2 (2002): 119–25

Kumar, Ambuj *et al.*, 'Are Experimental Treatments for Cancer in Children Superior to Established Treatments? Observational Study of Randomised Controlled Trials by the Children's Oncology Group', *British Medical Journal* 331 (December 2005): 1295

Kumar, Ambuj *et al.*, 'Evaluation of New Treatments in Radiation Oncology', *Journal of the American Medical Association* 293 (2005): 970–8

Kurlansky, Mark, *Salt*, 2002

Kurlansky, Mark, *The Big Oyster*, 2007

Lai, Timothy *et al.*, 'Is Ophthalmology Evidence Based?', *British Journal of Ophthalmology* 87 (2003):385–90

Lax, Eric, *The Mould in Dr Florey's Coat*, 2004

Lee, J. S. *et al.*, 'Is General Thoracic Surgical Practice Evidence Based?', *Annals of Thoracic Surgery* 70, 2 (August 2000): 429–31

Lewis, Frederic T., 'The Introduction of Biological Stains', *The Anatomical Record* 83, 2 (1942): 229–53 (Wiley-Liss)

Link, Karl Paul, 'The Discovery of Dicoumarol and Its Sequels', *Circulation* 19 (1959): 97–107

Livingstone, David, *Narrative of an Expedition to the Zambesi*, 1865, 2001 edn.

Loudon, Irvine, *The Use of Historical Controls and Concurrent Controls to Assess the Effects of Sulphonamides*, 1936–1945, 2002; the James Lind Library: www.jameslindlibrary.org [accessed Monday 8 October 2007]

Maclagan, T., 'The Treatment of Acute Rheumatism by Salicin', *Lancet* 1 (1876): 342–3 and 383–4

Malone, Dumas, *The Story of the Declaration of Independence*, 1954

Markham, Clements, *Travels in Peru and India*, 1862

Marks, Harry, *The Progress of Experiment*, 1997

Mather, H. *et al.*, 'Acute Myocardial Infarction: Home and Hospital Treatment', *British Medical Journal* 3 (1971): 334–8

Matzen, P., 'How Evidence-based is Medicine?' *Ugeskr Laeger* 165, 14 (31 March 2003): 1431–5 [Medline abstract only, the original Danish being beyond me]

Maynard, Alan and Chalmers, Iain (eds), *Non-random Reflections on Health Services Research*, 1997

McTavish, Janice Rae, *Pain and Profits*, 2004

Medical Research Council Therapeutic Trials Committee, 'The Serum Treatment of Lobar Pneumonia', *British Medical Journal* 1 (1934): 241–5

Meynell, G., 'John Locke and the Preface to Thomas Sydenham's *Observationes Medicae*', *Medical History* 50(1): 93–110, 2006

Michaud, G., 'Are Therapeutic Decisions Supported by Evidence from Health Care Research?', *Archives of Internal Medicine* 158, 15 (10–24 August 1998): 1665–8

Million Women Study Collaborators, 'Breast Cancer and Hormone-replacement Therapy in the Million Women Study', *Lancet* 362 (2003): 419–27

Miner, Jonathan and Hoffhines, Adam, 'The Discovery of Aspirin's Antithrombotic Effects', *Texas Heart Institute Journal* 34, 2 (2007): 179–86

Moncrieff, J., Wessely, S. and Hardy, R., 'Active Placebos Versus Antidepressants for Depression', Cochrane Database of Systematic Reviews 2004, issue 1, art. no. CD003012, DOI: 10.1002/14651858.CD003012.pub2

Moore, Thomas, *Deadly Medicine*, 1995

Morabia, Alfredo, *Pierre-Charles-Alexandre Louis and the evaluation of bloodletting* 2004; the James Lind Library: www.jameslindlibrary.org [accessed Monday 22 October 2007]

Morens, David, 'Death of a President', *New England Journal of Medicine* 341(9 December 1999): 1845–50

Mosteller, Frederick, 'Innovation and Evaluation', *Science* 211, 4485, (23 February 1981): 881–6

Nobel Lectures, *Physiology or Medicine 1922–1941*, 1965

North, Robert, 'Benjamin Rush, MD: Assassin or Beloved Healer?', *Baylor University Medical Center Proceedings* 13 (2000): 45–9

O'Brien, John, 'An in-vivo trial of an anti-adhesive drug', *Thrombosis et Diathesis Haemorrhagica*, 1963, 9: 120–25

O'Brien, John, 'Effects of salicylates on human platelets', *Lancet* 1968, April 13 ii (7546): 779–83

Osler, William, *The Principles and Practice of Medicine*, 1892

Osler, William and McCrae, Thomas, *The Principles and Practice of Medicine*, 1920

Pereira, Jonathan, 'Lectures on Materia Medica', *London Medical Gazette* (13 August 1836)

Pereira, Jonathan, *The Elements of Materia Medica and Therapeutics*, 1857

Perutz, Max, *I Wish I'd Made You Angry Earlier*, 2003

Peto, Richard, 'Possible Explanations for the Results of CRASH', *Lancet* 365 (2005): 213

Peto, Richard and Baigent, Colin, 'Trials: the Next 50 Years', *British Medical Journal* 317 (1998): 1170–1

Peto, Richard, Collins, Rory and Gray, Richard, 'Large-Scale Randomized Evidence', *Journal of Clinical Epidemiology* 48, 1 (1995): 23–40

Porter, Roy, *The Greatest Benefit to Mankind*, 1997

Potter, C. W., 'A History of Influenza', *Journal of Applied Microbiology* 91 (2001): 572–9

Rajkumar, S. Vincent, 'Thalidomide: Tragic Past and Promising Future', *Mayo Clinic Proceedings* 79, 7 (July 2004): 899–903

Rang, H. P. (ed), *Drug Discovery and Development*, 2006

Rocco, Fiammetta, *Quinine*, 2003

Rosenberg, William and Donald, Anna, 'Evidence Based Medicine', *British Medical Journal* 310 (1995): 1122–6

Royal Society of London, *Biographical Memoirs of the Royal Society of London*, 9 (1963): 91–120

Ryan, Frank, *Tuberculosis: The Greatest Story Never Told*, 1992

Siegel, Rudolph and Poynter, F. N. L., 'Robert Talbor, Charles II and Conchona, a Contemporary Document', *Medical History* 1 (6 January 1962): 82–5

Silverman, William, *Where's the Evidence?*, 1998

Silverman, William, 'The Schizophrenic Career of a "Monster Drug"', *Paediatrics* 110, 2 (August 2002): 404–6

Smith, Gordon and Pell, Jill, 'Parachute Use to Prevent Death and Major Trauma Related to Gravitational Challenge', *British Medical Journal* 327 (2003): 1459–61

Sneader, Walter, *Drug Discovery*, 2005

Stolberg, M., *Inventing the Randomized Double-blind Trial: The Nuremberg Salt Test of 1835*, 2006; the James Lind Library: www.jameslind library.org [accessed Wednesday 24 October 2007]

Streptomycin in Tuberculosis Trials Committee, 'Streptomycin Treatment of Pulmonary Tuberculosis', *British Medical Journal* 2 (1948): 769–82

Taubenberger, J. and Morens, D., '1918 Influenza: the Mother of All Pandemics', *Emerg. Infect. Dis.* 12, 1 (2006): 15–22

Thomas, Lewis, *The Fragile Species*, 1996

Thomson, Thomas, *A System of Chemistry*, 1817

Thomson, Thomas, *The History of Chemistry*, 1830

Thoreau, Henry David, *Civil Disobedience*, 1993

Tibi, S., *Al-Razi and Islamic Medicine in the 9th Century*, 2005; the James Lind Library: www.jameslindlibrary.org [accessed Thursday 25 October 2007]

Tsuruoka, Koki *et al.*, 'Drug Treatment in General Practice in Japan is Evidence Based', *British Medical Journal* 313 (1996): 114–5

Turner, Erick *et al.*, 'Selective Publication of Antidepressant Trials and Its Influence on Apparent Efficacy', *New England Journal of Medicine* 358 (2008): 252–60

Vastag, Brian, 'Medicine on the Lewis and Clark Trail', *Journal of the American Medical Association* 289 (2003): 1227–30

Vollmann, Jochen and Winau, Rolf, 'Informed Consent in Human Experimentation before the Nuremberg Code', *British Medical Journal* 313 (7 December 1996): 1445–7

Volmink, J., *The Willow as a Hottentot (Khoikhoi) Remedy for Rheumatic Fever*, 2005; the James Lind Library: www.jameslindlibrary.org [accessed Thursday 4 October 2007]

Wainwright, Milton, 'The History of the Therapeutic Use of Crude Penicillin', *Medical History* 31 (1987): 41–50

Wainwright, Milton and Swan, Harold, 'C. G. Paine and the Earliest Surviving Clinical Records of Penicillin Therapy', *Medical History* 30 (1986): 42–56

Warren, Kenneth and Mosteller, Frederick, *Doing More Good Than Harm*, 1993

Weizmann, Chaim, *Trial and error: The autobiography of Chaim Weizmann*, 1950

Whittington, Craig *et al.*, 'Selective Serotonin Reuptake Inhibitors in Childhood Depression: Systematic Review of Published versus Unpublished Data', *Lancet* 363 (2004): 1341–5

Wilson, James Grant and Fiske, John (eds), *Appleton's Cyclopædia of American Biography*, 1901

Witkop, Bernhard, 'Paul Ehrlich and His Magic Bullets – Revisited', *Proceedings of the American Philosophical Society* 143, 4 (December 1999) 540–57

Wittes, Robert E., 'Therapies for Cancer in Children – Past Successes, Future Challenges', *New England Journal of Medicine* 348 (February 2003): 747–9

Wolinsky, Howard, 'The Battle of Helsinki', *EMBO Reports, European Molecular Biology Organization* 7, 7 (2006): 670–2

Women's Health Initiative Investigators, 'Risks and Benefits of Estrogen Plus Progestin in Healthy Postmenopausal Women', *Journal of the American Medical Association* 288, 3 (17 July 2002): 321–33

Wootton, David, *Bad Medicine*, 2006

World Health Organisation, *Maternal Mortality in 2000*, 2004

Wright, Charles R. A., 'On the Action of Organic Acids and their Anhydrides on the Natural Alkaloids', *Journal of the Chemical Society* 27 (1874): 1031–43

Yates, David and Roberts, Ian, 'Corticosteroids in Head Injury', *British Medical Journal* 321 (2000): 128–9

Yates, Frank and Mather, Kenneth, 'Ronald Aylmer Fisher', *Biographical Memoirs of Fellows of the Royal Society of London* 9 (1963): 91–120

Yoshioka, Alan, 'Use of Randomisation in the Medical Research Council's Clinical Trial of Streptomycin in Pulmonary Tuberculosis in the 1940s', *British Medical Journal* 317 (1998): 1220–3

Acknowledgments

My thanks to Peter Buckman at Ampersand Agency, and especially to Jenny Uglow at Chatto & Windus for her generous editorial help. Iain Chalmers kindly contributed both time and suggestions, and the James Lind Library in which he has been so involved was a particularly good resource. Matthew Stephens of the University of Chicago answered several queries while I was working on this book, but his obvious enthusiasm for statistics, to which I was occasionally forced to listen years ago while hauling him up and down various branches of the Thames, was an even more useful lesson.

The impulse to write this book emerged gradually out of repeated exposure to both the theoretical and clinical difficulties involved in treating patients, and the questions that come up over the value of what a doctor has to offer. It was aided by the interest in evidence based medicine shown by so many of my teachers and colleagues, and sparked in particular by two wonderful books that I greatly recommend: William Silverman's *Where's the Evidence?* and David Wootton's *Bad Medicine*. It was also very much the result of repeated conversations over many years with Marion Mafham about the role of our shared medical work, as well as her involvement in a large-scale clinical trial. Our friend and neighbour Richard Lehman, particularly with his infectious interest in reading medical journals and considering their contents, has also been a tremendous influence.

This book omits many of the milestones in the development of evidence based medicine. My intention has not been to track them comprehensively, but to focus on those that were most influential or interesting. I will undoubtedly have missed some that I should have included, and mentioned a few that I would have been best off omitting. For these and any other errors I take full responsibility.

Index